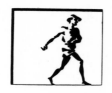

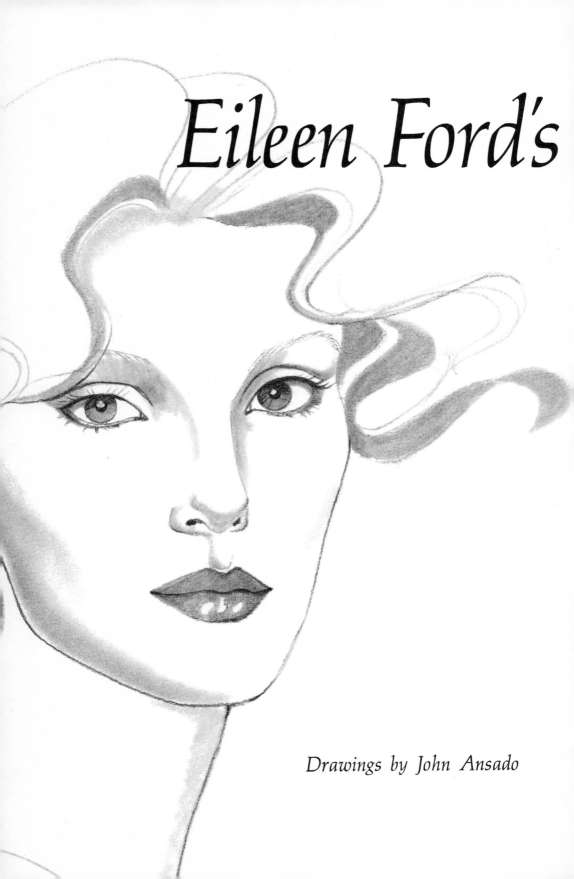

Eileen Ford's

Drawings by John Ansado

Beauty Now and Forever

SECRETS

OF BEAUTY AFTER 35

SIMON AND SCHUSTER / NEW YORK

Library of Congress Cataloging in Publication Data

Ford, Eileen.
  Eileen Ford's beauty now and forever.

  Includes index.
  1. Beauty, Personal.   2. Women—Health and
hygiene.   3. Middle age—Health and hygiene.   I.
Title.
RA778.7196   646.7'2'024041   76–56746
ISBN 0–671–22447–6

My thanks to Rochelle Larkin for all her research, and special thanks always to my agent, Roz Targ, who pressured me into finishing this book.

To my husband, Jerry, who cares

Contents

Introduction

The more I read, the more I travel, the more I see, the more I know that few teen-agers struggling for so-called identity face the real problems that those of us beyond thirty-five have to face. Somehow youth has the strength of youth to call on, it can look to the future. But those of us past thirty-five don't have that luxury of looking at the future—because it's here—right now.

It does not stand to reason that simply because one is mature, one is secure—that one's patterns for living and being are set; on the contrary, these are the years that perhaps open our eyes to the truth—and the truth is not always a pleasant thing. Economic security may not have been achieved in accordance with youthful expectations; marital security is all too often threatened at this stage of the game; it's a time for heart attacks, failing sexual powers and hysterectomies; and, to frost the cake, it's a time when anyone, man or woman, can look in a mirror and come to the dreadful realization that those "golden years" may not be so golden after all. These years may be the crisis years.

While my writing heretofore has largely been limited to

beauty, I've come to find that my world has grown larger than that. Traveling for my books *Eileen Ford's Book of Model Beauty, Secrets of the Model's World,* and *A More Beautiful You in 21 Days* has brought me in contact with literally thousands of people. After thirty years as an agent, I am still in contact with many of my former models. Everywhere I meet people looking for assurance—assurance and knowledge about themselves—and that's what this book is about: about you and your doubts, about your needs, physical and mental.

Heaven comes after we're dead, but that doesn't mean that life has to be purgatory before then. Life should be joyous—tempered by experiences that may sadden us, surely—but all in all, living should be much more pleasure than pain. It's just that somehow, as people mature, they start to see things in a truer light, and that can be frightening. All my adult years I've been too busy giving advice to give in to the insecurities that others face. But I realize that they are there, and now I've put together for you all this knowledge that I've acquired, to help give you insight into yourself and to help you find your own security.

This book is my most ambitious undertaking because I feel this almost desperate need on the part of everyone to have someone in whom they can confide and trust. I don't mean a psychiatrist or a lawyer or other professional person—I just mean a human being who can answer some questions, maybe about relationships with husbands or wives, or rejuvenating processes, or what have you. Just a person who has seen a lot and is willing to listen and discuss. I hope to be that person for you. For as I meet more and more of you, and like you—I feel that need and the will inside of me to try to help. I guess I should have had lots more than four children, because that's how I look at people who seem to need my advice—a whole large family is what you are to me; and what I'd like to do with this book is design for you a plan for living in the most joyous way possible. That my advice will encompass health and beauty is essential, because these two factors are all-important to your self-confidence and feeling of overall well-being. Armed with this essential knowledge, you will find it easier to face the other problems that are bound to arise, and arming yourself with just a little more knowledge and insight can make life totally enjoyable. There need not be any crisis years—just glorious, meaningful, rich years, looking your best, feeling your best and contributing to your enjoyment of every facet of the world around you!

1

The Crisis Years

Over the last years I've written a great deal about beauty for you. In *Eileen Ford's Book of Model Beauty*, I attempted to set out a general beauty program that every woman could follow from her teens to forever. In *A More Beautiful You in 21 Days*, I devised a quick-weight-loss, beauty and exercise program for those of you who are in dire need of instant rehabilitation. It is, incidentally, a sensational cookbook. The present book, *Eileen Ford's Beauty Now and Forever*, does, of course, deal with beauty—but more than that, it is about living. Today we seem to be caught in a perpetual maelstrom. We're hurried, pressured and harried to such a point that there doesn't seem to be any real person left. Where are we? Where did the years go? What happened to the loving, happy human beings that we were?

We all start our adult lives with anticipation—our hopes, our dreams, our physical beauty and forces are at their peak. How can anything go wrong? We love and are loved—happiness is a goal that we are all sure to achieve. The years go by so quickly that few of us notice the glitter wearing off. The pressures of married or business life or both close in—close in about us so tightly that we forget our lovely dreams and aspirations. What happened to the bright-eyed girl who was never going to let her husband see her without her makeup or with her hair in rollers? Where is the tender young husband whose every glance caused a shiver of anticipation? Was there a young mother who didn't mind the noise of a lot of children in the house? She's gone—and as the years pass, suddenly that bright-eyed girl takes a long look at herself—bulging stomach, back beginning to slump (if it hasn't done so already), hair askew. The children are in school and the husband is not looking in her direction the way he once did—and no wonder—for the girl of his dreams has arrived at the crisis years, and her neglected appearance, tears, constant fatigue and complaints tell him so. She doesn't have to say a word. He knows. They both forgot to make a real plan for the years when they would both pass thirty, forty, fifty, sixty and beyond, and they wake up too late to discover the beauty of living.

There really is a beauty to living life to its fullest. Life can pass us by all too quickly without a plan for the present and the future. To enjoy every minute, you've got to think about how you're going to do it. Looking our best, feeling our best, are part of living our best. It takes a little care and the time to give yourself that care. The good life is not just for someone else—it's for you. This book is to help you achieve it.

"It's easy for you," I can hear you say to me, "you live a rich and easy life." But do I? My schedule is this: Arise at seven, take my last at-home daughter to high school, work (and I mean work!) from eight thirty to six or seven. I entertain approximately four nights a week, run three homes, take six or seven quick business trips to Europe and several around the United States each year, write my books, plan meals, buy theater tickets, football tickets, make dentist and doctor appointments, deal with plumbers, painters and electricians, raise flowers, herbs and vegetables, care for two enormous dogs and myriad cats, plan two-week vacations with the family and do whatever else I have to. If you call that easy—try it.

But I do it because I must; it's a pattern of living that I myself set, and I'm stuck with it. Sometimes I mind it, lots; mostly I enjoy it because I've learned to live with it. The hardest part of it all, for me, has been learning to stay a woman—a well-groomed, good-figured woman who doesn't lose her sense of femininity. I may not be a geriatric sex symbol, but I try to appeal to my husband and to other men. I try not to give orders to Jerry, although I spend much of my business time giving orders. It has not been easy, but I've managed to learn and am glad that I did, for I can truthfully say I'm a happy woman.

It seems as though it were yesterday, or last week, or not so long, long ago, that I had our first child, Jamie, who is now thirty. She was followed by Billy, Katie and Lacey. The agency started with the birth of Jamie and grew along with the other three. It was only the other day that I was twenty-two; and it won't be long until someone is going to have to fit fifty-five candles on my cake and that I will be a grandmother!

My cup, it seemed to me, was running over; *all over* the place. For in spite of the frantic pace I keep, my husband seemed to be content (the years of learning to live together gone), the children were growing up and turning out even better than we dared hope. Business wasn't bad—so what could be amiss in my frantic little paradise? Nothing—until one day Jerry told me that the glasses I'd been wearing for twenty years looked terrible. I put away the offensive specs that had aroused such emotion in my beloved's normally placid breast and pulled out a comparatively new pair, only five or six years old. A few days later he told me that those were terrible, too. From a husband who ordinarily didn't notice much about me, that was a low blow. When he followed up a few days later by telling me my stockings sagged, when he wanted to stay in town to play tennis with friends on a Saturday morning instead of going to the country as planned, there was no longer any dodging what he was trying to tell me.

It happened that Jerry had made these criticisms at a time when I was beset by business worries. I developed a middle ear infection that made me so miserable I could hardly stand up. I was quite ready to leave the agency and my husband. I knew then that I had plunged into my crisis years.

What is a crisis year? I should really say "crisis years," and they begin sooner rather than later. Everyone's crisis years start at a different time. It's a time when marriages, bodies and people fall apart. It's a time of identity crisis, when one realizes that goals may have not been achieved, the things that you promised yourself and others didn't happen. The children are either grown or almost there, and there are almost or in fact more years passed by than lie ahead—which means that lots of plans may never be put into action. Menopause, female or male, may soon or currently have to be faced. One's whole life style is changing. For many of us, as we question our own drives, it is a time of self-searching and wondering. Glands may be in an uproar; certainly our minds may be. Your husband looks at you critically, wondering what happened to his girl; and maybe you look at his sagging tummy and wonder what happened to him, too. It can be a miserable time. That's why I call this transitory time "the crisis years."

When I say that these years are transitory, you have to believe me. They will pass. If you're in their midst, you really know what I'm talking about. If you haven't quite reached them or are just about to, you can thank heaven that you've picked up this book. One way or the other, this book is about living through a time when we should all be beginning to be, or are, settled down. It is an explanation of what happens and how to live through these times. It takes determination on your part—you've got to make up your mind that you are not going to let things slide, or to give up entirely. A woman need *not* have lines of discontent and neglect on her face, nor a man a scowl level that portrays the same condition.

There is nothing so precious as a well-adjusted mind and body. You've got to avoid the pitfalls of bad health, bad beauty habits and lack of physical regimen, which are so detrimental to the real art of living—the beauty of living.

The following chapters will tell you what I feel you must do in order to live your life to its most delicious fullest. It's not difficult, so why not try it? You'll feel and look so good that you'll bounce through each day happy, cheerful and healthy. You'll never know or remember there was a crisis year at all.

2

The Super Fourteen-Day
Diet and Exercise Program

I guess I'm like an accordion; I go from overweight back into shape so many times that to me it's a miracle that I can ever get back to where I started. But I do, and I do because when I find I've slipped, I just start all over again.

I've tried every kind of diet that man can try and survive, some with more success than others. Recently it's been very "in" to be a vegetarian. I've noticed that all vegetarians are very thin. I've noticed, too, that their skin color is pallid. After giving a great deal of thought to the subject I finally decided that it certainly couldn't hurt if I tried being a vegetarian for two weeks, so I did and it worked! I lost inches and inches and pounds and pounds. I combined the vegetarian diet with an old theory of mine: *No liquid one-half hour before, during or after meals.*

To those of you used to a glass of wine with dinner, or those who drink gallons of water with your meals, this may mean a radical shift in your thinking. But change never hurt anyone, and in this case, change did this anyone a great deal of good— so much so that I don't drink liquids with my meals at all any more. When I think of my beautiful wine cellar full of some of the best wines I've been able to acquire, I often feel a twinge of regret; but vanity has me in its clutches so I just don't give in, and as far as Jerry is concerned, there's just that much more wine for him!

If you've read any of my other books, you know that I like to eat more than somewhat. The vision of just plain vegetables doesn't appeal to me *at all!* In fact, I know very well that had I started my vegetarian diet that way, I might have lasted a whole forty-eight hours. So I looked around for recipes for vegetables that would, hopefully, slim me and at the same time satisfy the gourmet urge that is so strong in me. There are so many recipes in my files that the fourteen days were fun. Tomatoes provençal, carrots vichy, spinach with onion, fried cabbage, baked, stuffed, sautéed zucchini—the list was endless. I've put it together for you in a fourteen-day diet-and-recipe combination. It isn't just good, it is sublime. Also, it includes the kind of vitamins I took as a supplement and a gentle reminder not to drink liquids one-half hour before or after meals, and, above all, during them. This means that if you're going to get in those eight glasses of liquid that we need daily, it has to be *between* meals!

The other thing to bear in mind is that large portions are a catastrophe because they increase our capacity for food. To lose weight, it is essential to take smaller portions (that is if you are a big eater). It's also far better to eat five or six small portions a day than one or two big ones. In order for you to stay on this diet, I am going to give you six rules of diet that you can use now and forever. Always remember them.

1. Eat the freshest fruits and vegetables—they are more nutritious and appetizing.

2. Never let yourself get hungry. Keep snacks handy in the refrigerator: carrots, celery, watercress, cucumbers and raw mushrooms. Hunger pains diminish willpower drastically.

3. Eat small amounts of food at a time to "shrink your stomach." Five small meals a day are better than one enormous one.

4. Use a pepper mill, lemon juice and herbs to help give your food flavor. Try to cut down on salt. Salt helps your body to retain water and therefore weight.

5. Weigh yourself every day at about the same time.

6. Stand in front of a mirror, stripped down, every day and believe that you are thinner, if only by an eighth of a pound.

Every day I took 1,000 units of vitamin C, a multipurpose vitamin and ⅓ cup of Gevral protein mixed with a glass of fresh grapefruit juice. You can buy dried protein in most health-food stores. There are about 100 calories in the protein alone, so it makes a very good breakfast combined with the fresh juice.

Lunch has to be light. For those of us who work, it's often hard to get out of the office—so lunch may well have to be imported by the eater, in which case, just plain raw vegetables with salt and pepper are satisfying. If you are lucky enough to be home for lunch, make it a salad. I'm going to provide you with fourteen different salads for your lunchtime. You'll probably never be hungry, but if you are, turn to the crisp celery, cucumber and carrot sticks that you must keep in the refrigerator—or raw mushrooms, which contain practically no calories!

You'll see that I've named lots of these recipes after friends and models who have been with us over the years. It is my salute to them for their continuing beauty as they graduate from Ford to their wonderful lives of today.

A diet must be judged by its results. The results of this one are surefire. What have you got to lose in fourteen days? I'll tell you what! Weight, weight, weight—and excess inches all over your body, since the diet is combined with special exercises. You will lose whatever excess you see in the mirror. This is what you want; and you can have it with just about no effort. I did it; you can do it. Your children, if still at home, will approve; your husband will not only love the food; he will love the newly shaped woman he is sharing those vegetarian dinners with. However, before you embark on any kind of diet, check with your doctor. More likely than not, he'll encourage you to shed that extra poundage, but ask first. *Further, when you do diet, don't follow this regime for more than fourteen days.* If you follow it faithfully, you will find that you have lost a reasonable amount of weight. You may even have helped re-shape your figure—if you've done the exercises. Still, two weeks at a time is enough.

You'll do fourteen minutes of exercise a day to go with your diet. Imagine—only fourteen minutes of exercise to reshape the body. This new body can be maintained easily with the diet-and-exercise maintenance program devised especially for you in the following chapters.

Start off with a bang for the first fourteen days and continue at your own pace with the maintenance program. Write me, tell me of your success; I'm yearning to hear from you!

DAY 1

MENU

Breakfast

> 1,000 units vitamin C
> 1 multipurpose vitamin pill that contains minerals
> 1 cup of freshly squeezed grapefruit juice combined with
> ⅓ cup Gevral protein supplement.

Lunch

> Salad—Lauren Hutton
> with French Dressing

Dinner

> Panama Consommé
> Alana Hamilton's Stuffed Artichokes
> String Bean Salad—Candice Bergen
> Ratatouille Cappucine

• *Salad—Lauren Hutton*

> *1¼ green peppers, cut into little sticks*
> *½ very small green cabbage, shredded*
> *½ very small red cabbage, shredded*
> *½ medium cauliflower, broken into flowerets*
> *1 young cucumber, sliced*
> *3 young scallions, chopped*
> *1 celery heart, chopped*
> *2 tomatoes, peeled, seeded, and cut into eighths*
> *¼ head escarole*
> *¼ head Boston lettuce*
> *¼ large head Romaine*
> *¼ garlic clove*
> *1 teaspoon chopped chives*
> *¼ tablespoon chopped fresh dill*

Wash the vegetables before cutting, shredding or chopping as indicated above. Separate salad greens into leaves and wash them well. Put the greens and all the vegetables except the tomatoes in a bowl with lots of cracked ice until time to serve. Then drain and dry all the ingredients and place them in a large wooden bowl that has been well rubbed with cut garlic clove. Add the tomatoes. Sprinkle the chives and dill over the salad. Pour the French dressing over all. Toss well and serve. Serves 3 or 4.

French Dressing

> *½ tablespoon prepared mustard*
> *¾ teaspoon salt*
> *¼ cup tarragon wine vinegar*
> *¼ teaspoon freshly ground black pepper*
> *1 tablespoon sour cream*

Place mustard in a bowl, stir in salt. Beat in vinegar with a wire whisk (a tablespoon of water at this point is helpful for texture), add pepper and stir in sour cream.

• *Panama Consommé*

> *Combine and heat the contents of:*
> *1 can condensed consommé*
> *1 can condensed madrilène*
> *Stir in:*
> *The juice of 1 large orange. Serve chilled "on the rocks."*
> *Serves 4.*

• *Ratatouille Cappucine*

> *Put in a deep skillet or heavy casserole:*
> *¼ cup salad oil*
> *Sauté until golden:*
> *⅜ cup thinly sliced onions*
> *2 cloves garlic chopped fine*
> *Remove the onions and garlic from the casserole and combine in layers with:*
> *2 cups zucchini, diced*
> *1 cup peeled, seeded, quartered tomatoes*
> *1½ cups peeled, diced eggplant*
> *Add to each layer: salt and pepper*

Sprinkle the top with small amount of salad oil. Simmer, covered, over very low heat 35 to 45 minutes. Uncover and continue to heat 10 minutes longer to reduce the amount of liquid. Serve hot or cold. Serves 4.

• *Alana Hamilton's Stuffed Artichokes*

> *4 medium artichokes*
> *3 cups chopped parsley*

2 cloves garlic, finely chopped
1 teaspoon salt
⅛ teaspoon freshly ground black pepper
½ teaspoon oregano
Juice of ½ lemon
1 tablespoon salad oil

Prepare the artichokes for stuffing by removing the center fuzzy part and tiny inner leaves. Preheat oven to moderate—350° F. Combine the parsley, garlic, salt, pepper and oregano and pack into the center of each artichoke. Arrange the artichokes in a baking dish just large enough to accommodate them snugly, or, if the pan is larger, tie each with a string to retain its shape. To the dish add boiling water to the depth of 1 inch. Drizzle the lemon juice and oil over the artichokes. Cover and bake 30 to 45 minutes. Cool to room temperature before serving. Serve topped with thin lemon wedges. Serves 4.

• *String Bean Salad—Candice Bergen*

1 package frozen whole green beans
½ cup beef bouillon
¼ teaspoon powdered dill
1 tablespoon finely chopped onions
⅛ cup French dressing
½ tablespoon Roquefort or blue cheese (optional)

After defrosting the beans in a colander, put them in a saucepan with the bouillon, dill and onions. When the liquid comes to a boil, lower the heat. Simmer for about 15 minutes, uncovered, by which time all the liquid should be absorbed. Watch carefully to avoid scorching. Remove the beans from the heat, add the dressing and the crumbled Roquefort or blue cheese, if desired. Mix well and marinate for 15 minutes. Serve without chilling further. Serves 4.

DAY 2

MENU

Breakfast

    1,000 units vitamin C
    1 multipurpose vitamin pill that contains minerals
    1 cup of freshly squeezed grapefruit juice combined with
        ⅓ cup Gevral protein supplement.

Lunch

    Salade de Champignons—Karen Graham

Dinner

    Galya Milovskaya's Blender Borscht
    Puree of leeks—Eileen's Favorite
    Spinach with Tomatoes—Mme. Chesnutt
    Sautéed Peppers—Jolly Earl

• *Salade de Champignons—Karen Graham*

Peel 12 large, firm white mushrooms. Slice thin, including stems, if firm and fresh. Season with 1 tablespoon lemon juice, 2 tablespoons sour cream and 1 tablespoon freshly grated horseradish. For larger quantities of mushrooms follow the same proportions: 2 parts sour cream to 1 part lemon juice and 1 part horseradish. Mix gently but well. Serve on a Boston lettuce leaf. Sprinkle with finely chopped parsley. Serves 4.

• *Galya Milovskaya's Blender Borscht*

> 2 cups tomato juice
> 2 cups canned beets
> 3 small dill pickles
> 3 tablespoons finely grated onion
> 1 drop hot pepper sauce
> 1 clove minced garlic

Combine all ingredients briefly in blender. Chill the soup and serve garnished with thinly sliced hard-boiled egg slices, diet sour cream, chopped fresh dill or fennel. Serves 4.

• *Puree of Leeks—Eileen's Favorite*

Prepare and cook until tender 6 leeks. Drain them well, chop them coarsely and put in blender to puree. For each cup add 2 tablespoons margarine, salt and pepper to taste. Stir and simmer them gently until blended. Serve the puree very hot with finely chopped parsley as garnish. Serves 4.

• *Spinach with Tomatoes—Mme. Chesnutt*

Cook until barely done 1 pound spinach. Drain and blend or chop fine. Add 6 to 8 tablespoons Italian tomato sauce or tomato puree.

Sauté 1 pressed clove garlic or 3 tablespoons minced onion in 3 or 4 tablespoons salad oil. Add the spinach-tomato mixture and correct the seasoning. Serves 3 or 4.

• *Sautéed Peppers—Jolly Earl*

> 1 clove garlic
> 6 tablespoons salad oil
> 4 green peppers seeded and finely sliced

1 teaspoon salt
1 teaspoon dried red pepper

Heat garlic in oil and fry until brown. Remove garlic and add peppers and seasonings. Sauté the peppers until they are limp. Remove with a slotted spoon. These may be served hot or cold. Serves 4.

DAY 3

MENU

Breakfast

> 1,000 units vitamin C
> 1 multipurpose vitamin pill that contains minerals
> 1 cup of freshly squeezed grapefruit juice combined with
> ⅓ cup of Gevral protein supplement.

Lunch

> Lala's Salade de Romaine

Dinner

> Spinach-Stuffed Tomatoes—Susan Blakely
> Puree of Broccoli—Tippi Hedren
> Baked Eggplant Slices as served by Robert Evans

• *Lala's Salade de Romaine*
(Romaine salad with anchovies and cheese)

> *1 clove garlic*
> *1 teaspoon salt*
> *½ teaspoon white pepper*
> *1 tablespoon wine vinegar*

½ teaspoon Dijon mustard
2 medium anchovy fillets
2 tablespoons salad oil
1 teaspoon grated onion
2 eggs, boiled 2 minutes
½ teaspoon chopped sweet basil
1 large head Romaine lettuce, cleaned and soaked in
    cold water ¾ hour, dried, cut in 4-inch lengths
1 tablespoon grated Parmesan cheese

Crush the garlic in a wooden salad bowl with the salt and pepper. Add the vinegar and mustard and mix. Mash the anchovies with these ingredients. Stir in the oil. Add the onion, eggs and basil and mix well. Add the Romaine, sprinkle with cheese and mix well, but gently. Serves 4.

• *Spinach-Stuffed Tomatoes—Susan Blakely*

¾ cup salad oil
½ cup pine nuts (pignoli)
2 medium onions, finely chopped
2 cloves garlic, finely chopped
1 pound spinach, cooked briefly, thoroughly drained,
    squeezed as dry as possible and finely chopped
salt and freshly ground black pepper to taste
4 medium tomatoes
dried or fresh basil to taste

Preheat oven to moderate 350° F.

In a skillet heat ¼ cup of the oil with the pine nuts and sauté nuts until lightly browned. Remove nuts and set aside. In the same pan, sauté the onions and garlic and cook briefly until the onions are pale golden in color. Remove from the heat.

Add the prepared spinach, the reserved nuts, ¼ cup of the remaining oil, the salt and pepper. Cut the stem ends from the tomatoes; hollow tomatoes out and sprinkle the insides with salt, pepper and a pinch of basil. Stuff the tomatoes with the spinach, place in a baking pan and pour the remaining oil over them. Bake until the tomatoes wrinkle, about 15 minutes. Chill. At serving time, bring up to room temperature. Serves 4.

• Puree of Broccoli—Tippi Hedren

Prepare and cook until just tender 1 bunch broccoli. Drain it well. Place in blender and puree. For each cup add 2 tablespoons margarine, salt and pepper. Stir and simmer gently until blended. Serve the puree very hot , garnished with finely chopped parsley. Serves 4.

• Baked Eggplant Slices as Served by Robert Evans

Preheat oven to 400° F. Pare 1 medium eggplant. Cut crosswise into slices ½ inch thick. Spread the slices on both sides with a mixture of salad oil and margarine. Season with salt and pepper to taste, grated onion, lemon juice and basil. Place eggplant slices on a baking sheet and bake until tender, about 12 minutes, turning them once. Garnish with chopped parsley or chervil. Serves 3 or 4.

DAY 4

MENU

Breakfast

> 1,000 units vitamin C
> 1 multipurpose vitamin pill that contains minerals
> 1 cup of freshly squeezed grapefruit juice combined with
>   ⅓ cup Gevral protein supplement

Lunch

> Chef's Salad—*Jack David*

Dinner

Fried Parsley Served All Over Paris
Zucchini and Mushroom Casserole—Melanie Griffith
Cauliflower Signorina Ascevedo
Green Beans—Ali MacGraw

• *Chef's Salad—Jack David*

1 clove garlic
1 tablespoon salt
1 teaspoon white pepper
1 teaspoon Dijon Mustard
dash Worcestershire sauce
1 tablespoon tomato puree
1 tablespoon wine vinegar
2 tablespoons salad oil
1 teaspoon each chopped fresh tarragon, parsley, chives
assorted salad greens (amount depending on how many
  people)
1 hard-boiled egg, thinly sliced
3 ounces Gruyère cheese, cut in julienne strips
3 ounces Swiss cheese, cut in julienne strips
8 capers

Crush the garlic clove against side of a wooden bowl with a wooden salad spoon. Add the salt, pepper, mustard, Worcestershire sauce and tomato puree; mix thoroughly. Pour in the vinegar, then the oil; mix in the chopped herbs. When well blended, add the salad greens and toss well with a wooden salad fork and spoon. Add the egg, Gruyère cheese, Swiss cheese and capers and toss again. Serve immediately.

• *Fried Parsley Served All Over Paris*

To retain crispness and color, have at least 2 to 3 inches of oil per cup of parsley, and bring the oil just to the smoking point in a deep, heavy saucepan. The parsley must be stemmed, washed and patted between towels until absolutely dry. Put in a frying basket 1 cup parsley prepared as above. Immerse the basket in the hot cooking oil and leave it 1 to 2 minutes. Remove basket. Drain parsley on paper towels. Serve immediately.

• Cauliflower Signorina Ascevedo

1 small head cauliflower
1 stick melted margarine

Parboil cauliflower in boiling salted water until barely tender. Remove from water and drain. Place cauliflower in a Pyrex baking dish. Pour over it the margarine. Place under a broiler for 5 minutes. (When you don't have to diet, mix the margarine with browned breadcrumbs and pat mixture on the cauliflower before putting under broiler.) Serves 4.

• Zucchini and Mushroom Casserole—Melanie Griffith

1½ pounds zucchini, trimmed and scrubbed
pinch of fresh chopped or dried dill
1 clove garlic
boiling salted water
½ pound mushrooms, sliced
3 tablespoons margarine
1 cup sour cream

Cut the zucchini crosswise into 1-inch slices, add the dill and garlic and boiling salted water to cover, and return to a boil. Reduce the heat, cover and simmer gently for 5 minutes, until the zucchini is tender; drain, reserving two tablespoons of the cooking liquid. Discard the garlic.

Sauté the mushrooms 5 minutes in the margarine, stirring occasionally. Add the sour cream, zucchini and reserved cooking liquid, stirring constantly. Correct the seasoning and heat thoroughly, but do not allow to boil.

Transfer the mixture to a casserole. Brown quickly under high broiler heat. Serves 4.

• *Green Beans—Ali MacGraw*

> *½ cup olive oil*
> *1 onion, sliced thin*
> *1 cup canned Italian plum tomatoes*
> *½ cup green pepper, chopped*
> *½ cup chopped celery*
> *¼ cup water*
> *1 teaspoon salt*
> *¼ teaspoon freshly ground black pepper*
> *2 cloves*
> *1 bay leaf*
> *6 sprigs parsley*
> *½ teaspoon dried chervil*
> *1 pound green beans, cooked until barely tender and drained*

In a skillet heat the oil, add the onion and cook until soft and golden brown. Add the tomatoes, green pepper, celery, water, salt and pepper. Tie the cloves, bay leaf, parsley and chervil in a small cheesecloth bag and add to the vegetables. Simmer, uncovered, about 25 minutes. Add the beans and continue simmering until the beans are heated through. Remove the spice bag and serve. Serves 4.

DAY 5

MENU

Breakfast

> 1,000 units vitamin C
> 1 multipurpose vitamin pill that contains minerals
> 1 cup of freshly squeezed grapefruit juice combined with
> ⅓ cup Gevral protein supplement

Lunch

> Artichoke Bottoms with Asparagus à la Pancho Auer with
>   Vinaigrette Sauce

Dinner

> Celery Braised in Consommé à la Lily Schulte
> Stuffed Zucchini—Iris Ory
> Red Cabbage Senta Berger

• *Artichoke Bottoms with Asparagus à la Pancho Auer*

> *4 cooked artichoke bottoms—canned can be used*
> *1 bunch cooked green asparagus tips—canned, if neces-*
>   *sary*
> *4 medium Boston lettuce leaves*
> *Vinaigrette Sauce (below)*
> *1 tablespoon chopped parsley*

Place the artichoke bottoms on the lettuce leaves. Fill with the Vinaigrette sauce. Cut up the asparagus tips and place over the artichokes. Sprinkle with parsley before serving. Serves 4.

Vinaigrette Sauce

This dressing may be made ahead and kept in the refrigerator or a cool place. It keeps indefinitely.

> *1 tablespoon Dijon mustard*
> *1 teaspoon salt*
> *dash freshly ground black pepper*
> *2 tablespoons water*
> *2 tablespoons wine vinegar*
> *2 tablespoons salad oil*

In a wooden salad bowl put mustard, salt, pepper and vinegar; blend thoroughly. Now blend in the salad oil and water a little at a time. (For garlic dressing, crush garlic clove against the inside of the wooden bowl with a wooden salad spoon; press it into the salt and pepper, so the garlic will completely blend into the dressing.) Herbs of your choice can be added, but do this last.

• Celery Braised with Consommé à la Lily Schulte

> 4 small bunches of celery or 2 large
> 1 cup consommé
> 2 tablespoons butter
> 1 small onion, minced
> 2 tablespoons flour
> paprika

Cut off part of the celery leaves. Cook the stalks whole, covered, in the consommé until tender. Remove the celery and keep warm. Reserve the broth. Heat the butter in a saucepan, add the onion and sauté, stirring, until transparent. Blend in the flour. Gradually add the broth and cook, stirring until thickened. Place the celery on a plate and cover with sauce. Sprinkle with paprika and serve at once. Serves 4.

• Stuffed Zucchini—Iris Ory

> 4 small zucchini, cut in half lengthwise
> salad oil
> 1 clove garlic, finely chopped
> 4 black olives, chopped (preferably soft type)
> ¾ tablespoon capers
> ¾ tablespoon chopped parsley
> 4 to 6 anchovy fillets, coarsely chopped
> breadcrumbs

Scoop out and discard seeds and a small amount of flesh from the zucchini. Sauté halves quickly in salad oil. Then parboil 5 to 10 minutes. Cool. Sauté the garlic in 2 tablespoons oil for 2 minutes. Add the chopped olives, capers, parsley, anchovies. Stuff the zucchini with this mixture, sprinkle with crumbs and brush with oil. Arrange the stuffed zucchini in a baking dish and bake in a 375° F. oven for 20 minutes, brushing once again with oil after 10 minutes of baking. Serve warm or at room temperature. Serves 4.

• Tomatoes Creole à la Ermine Ford

>2 tablespoons margarine
>4 large, skinned, sliced, seeded tomatoes or 1½ cups
>   canned tomatoes
>1 large minced onion
>2 tablespoons minced celery
>1 shredded green pepper
>¾ teaspoon salt
>¼ teaspoon paprika
>¼ teaspoon curry powder

Melt the margarine in a saucepan. Add the tomatoes, onion, celery and green pepper. Cook vegetables until they are tender, about 12 minutes. Add salt, pepper and curry powder. Stir well. Strain the juice from the vegetables and add to it enough diet sour cream to make 1½ cups of liquid. Mix gently over low heat to blend. Return vegetables to sauce to heat through but do not allow liquid to boil. Serves 4.

• Red Cabbage—Senta Berger

>1 small head of red cabbage
>2 tart red apples, cored but not peeled
>2 tablespoons bacon fat or lard
>salt and freshly ground black pepper to taste
>3 tablespoons vinegar
>1 teaspoon sugar

Remove the outer leaves of the cabbage and discard. Quarter, core and grate the cabbage.

Slice the cored, unpeeled apples into a skillet or saucepan and add the cabbage. Add the fat, salt and pepper and bring to a boil with just enough water to cover. Cover, reduce the heat and simmer until tender but still crisp, about fifteen minutes. Drain, reserving the liquid. Mix the vinegar and sugar in a saucepan and stir in the reserved liquid. Cook, stirring, until somewhat reduced. Add the drained cabbage, mix and reheat to serve. Serves 4.

DAY 6

MENU

Breakfast

> 1,000 units vitamin C
> 1 multipurpose vitamin pill that contains minerals
> 1 cup of freshly squeezed grapefruit juice combined with
>   ⅓ cup Gevral protein supplement.

Lunch

> Hearts of Palm with Anchovy Dressing—Joanne Dabney

Dinner

> Artichoke Bottoms with Mushroom Sauce—Nan Rees
> Rumanian Ghivetch à la Nina Blanchard
> Chicory and Orange Salad with Herb Dressing—
>   Lisa Penn

• *Hearts of Palm with Anchovy Dressing—Joanne Dabney*

> *1 can hearts of palm, drained*

Dressing:

> *2 cloves garlic*
> *½ teaspoon salt*
> *pinch white pepper*
> *2 ounces anchovy fillets (1 small can)*
> *1 hard-boiled egg yolk*
> *2 tablespoons vinegar*
> *1 teaspoon Dijon mustard*

¼ cup salad oil
1 teaspoon chopped parsley

Crush the garlic cloves with the salt and pepper in a wooden salad bowl. Add the anchovies and crush them against the wall of the bowl. Add the egg yolk and mix well to obtain a paste. Add vinegar to bowl. Stirring mixture with a wooden spoon, slowly add the mustard, the salad oil and finally the chopped parsley. Place the hearts of palm on a lettuce leaf for each portion and serve with dressing poured over. Serves 3 or 4.

• *Artichoke Bottoms with Mushroom Sauce—Nan Rees*

4 large artichokes, or use canned artichoke bottoms
chicken stock or salted water 2 inches deep when arti-
*   chokes are in pan*
1 tablespoon butter
1 tablespoon olive oil
⅛ pound mushrooms, diced
salt and freshly ground black pepper to taste
dried tarragon to taste
½ egg yolk, lightly beaten
½ tablespoon lemon juice

Cut off the top quarter of the artichokes and remove stems and tough outer leaves. Cook in the stock until tender, 20 minutes or longer. Remove the remaining leaves, saving them for another purpose, and, with a spoon, remove the prickly choke, leaving only the bottoms. If using canned, drain, rinse and pat dry.

In a skillet heat the butter and oil, add the mushrooms and cook until almost tender. Season with salt, pepper and tarragon. Add egg yolk and lemon juice. Blend thoroughly over low heat until thickened but do not boil. Arrange the artichoke bottoms on a serving platter and spoon the mushroom sauce over them.

• Rumanian Ghivetch à la Nina Blanchard

> ¼ head cauliflower, separated into flowerets
> 1 carrot, sliced thin
> ½ unpeeled eggplant, cubed
> ½ can (17-ounce size) Italian plum tomatoes, drained
> ¼ unpeeled yellow squash, sliced thin
> 1 medium onion, quartered
> ¼ cup green beans, cut into 2-inch slices
> ½ green or red pepper, seeded and sliced thin
> 1 stalk celery, cut fine
> salt and freshly ground black pepper to taste
> ¾ cup bouillon
> ¼ cup salad oil
> 1 clove garlic, crushed
> ¼ tablespoon chopped fresh dill or parsley

Preheat oven to moderate (350° F.). Arrange the vegetables in layers in a 2- to 3-quart ungreased casserole and sprinkle each layer with salt and pepper. Heat together the bouillon, salad oil and garlic. Add to the casserole. Sprinkle the dill over the top. Cover the casserole and bake until all the vegetables are tender, 1 hour or longer. Serve lukewarm. Serves 3 or 4.

• Chicory and Orange Salad with Herb Dressing— Lisa Penn

> 1 large head of chicory
> ⅓ celery heart, cut in julienne strips
> 1 small bunch of beets, cooked and grated
> 2 navel oranges
> Herb Dressing (see below)

Use only the white heart of the chicory, separated into 4 pieces, reserving the green leaves for another occasion (they may be cooked and pureed like spinach). Place 1 piece of chicory heart on each salad plate and arrange little heaps of julienned celery and grated beets over the chicory.

Carefully peel and seed the oranges and divide them into skinless sections. Arrange orange sections around each salad. Pour well-mixed herb dressing over all. Serves 4.

Herb Dressing

> *1 egg, hard-boiled*
> *⅓ cup sesame oil*
> *¼ cup lemon juice*
> *½ teaspoon mild prepared mustard*
> *1 teaspoon mixed dried fines herbes or 2 tablespoons fresh*
> *salt and freshly ground black pepper*

Chop the hard-boiled egg and mix with the oil, lemon juice, mustard, and salt and pepper to taste. Add the *fines herbes*. These may be a mixture of chervil, tarragon, parsley, and basil in proportions to taste; or other herbs may be used. Stir in the herbs and shake the dressing well.

DAY 7

MENU

Breakfast

> 1,000 units vitamin C
> 1 multipurpose vitamin pill that contains minerals
> 1 cup of freshly squeezed grapefruit juice combined with
> ⅓ cup Gevral protein supplement.

Lunch

> Boston Lettuce with Roquefort Dressing—Ingrid
> Boulting

Dinner

> Trini's Sardinian Salad with Dressing
> Sautéed Mushrooms—Maude Adams
> Braised Lettuce—Louella Boykin
> Italian Spinach—Elsa Martinelli

• *Boston Lettuce with Roquefort Dressing— Ingrid Boulting*

> *1 or 2 heads of Boston lettuce, washed, separated into leaves and dried*

Dressing:

> *1 teaspoon salt*
> *½ teaspoon white pepper*
> *1 teaspoon Dijon mustard*
> *1 tablespoon white wine vinegar*
> *2 tablespoons salad oil*
> *½ teaspoon grated horseradish*
> *2 tablespoons Roquefort cheese*
> *1 tablespoon sour cream*

Place lettuce leaves, broken into serving-size pieces, in a wooden salad bowl. In another small, deep bowl, mix the salt, pepper and mustard thoroughly. Add the vinegar, mix well. Add the oil slowly. Add the horseradish and last, the Roquefort cheese, crumbled fine, together with the sour cream. The dressing should be quite smooth. For best flavor, do not chill dressing, unless it has to stand for several hours. Pour immediately over salad, mix and serve at once. Serves 4.

• Trini's Sardinian Salad with Dressing

> 1 small mozzarella cheese, chopped
> 4 hard-boiled eggs, chopped
> 2 bunches parsley, chopped
> 1½ pounds ripe tomatoes, diced and seeded
> 1 head Romaine washed, dried and broken into pieces,
>   coarse veins removed
> a good handful fresh mint or basil, or a combination of
>   the two
> 2 medium onions, chopped

Mix all the ingredients in a salad bowl and serve with dressing below. Serves 4.

Dressing:

> juice of 2 lemons
> 6 teaspoons salad oil
> 2 generous pinches each of salt and pepper

Mix well before adding to salad.

• Sautéed Mushrooms—Maude Adams

> 1 pound mushrooms
> 2 tablespoons margarine
> 1 tablespoon cooking oil
> 1 clove garlic

Prepare mushrooms for cooking by washing or peeling. Use caps alone or caps and stems sliced to uniform thickness. Melt the margarine and cooking oil over moderately high heat until a haze forms. Add the mushrooms, shaking the pan so that the mushrooms are coated with fat but not scorched. Drop in the garlic clove. Continue to cook over moderately high heat, shaking the pan frequently. At first the mushrooms will seem dry and will almost imperceptibly absorb the fat. In a few minutes they will release their moisture. Continue to shake the pan now and then for 3 to 5 minutes, depending on the size of the mushroom pieces. Remove the garlic. Serve at once. Serves 4.

• Braised Lettuce—Louella Boykin

> *4 small heads Boston lettuce*
> *boiling salted water*
> *melted margarine*
> *2 tablespoons finely chopped onion*
> *2 tablespoons finely chopped carrot*
> *1 cup beef stock or canned consommé*
> *salt and freshly ground black pepper to taste*
> *chopped parsley*

Preheat oven to moderate (325° F.). Wash lettuce and cook, covered, in a small amount of boiling salted water 2 minutes. Drain and press out remainder of moisture lightly with a dry cloth. Cut each head in half. Margarine the bottom of a casserole and sprinkle with the chopped onion and carrot. Tuck the tops of the lettuce under and place flat on top of the vegetables. Add the stock and sprinkle with salt and pepper.

Cover with aluminum foil and bake 45 minutes. Transfer the lettuce to a warm serving dish and keep hot. Reduce the liquid in the casserole and pour over the lettuce. Before serving, sprinkle with parsley and additional melted margarine. Serves 4.

• Italian Spinach—Elsa Martinelli

> *2 pounds spinach, well washed and trimmed*
> *3 tablespoons margarine*
> *4 tablespoons salad oil*
> *1 clove garlic, finely chopped*
> *salt to taste*
> *¼ teaspoon cayenne pepper*
> *coarsely grated Parmesan cheese*

Cut the spinach into coarse shreds. Drop into boiling salted water to cover and boil 30 seconds. Drain well and place in a baking dish. In a skillet, heat the margarine and oil. Add the garlic, salt and cayenne and sauté over low heat 5 minutes. Combine the oil mixture with the spinach and sprinkle with cheese and a little additional melted margarine. Brown quickly under a broiler. Serves 4 generously.

DAY 8

MENU

Breakfast

> 1,000 units vitamin C
> 1 multipurpose vitamin pill that contains minerals
> 1 cup of freshly squeezed grapefruit juice combined with
> ⅓ cup of Gevral protein supplement.

Lunch

> Orange and Mint Salad—Jean Shrimpton

Dinner

> Blender Gazpacho—Suzy Parker
> Boiled Artichokes Vinaigrette—Heather Bernard
> Zucchini in a Pan alla Signora Piazzi
> Red Cabbage with Apples—Trice Tomsen

• *Orange and Mint Salad—Jean Shrimpton*

Peel as many large navel oranges as desired, removing all white pith. Slice, discarding ends, and arrange in overlapping slices on plates. Sprinkle with finely chopped fresh mint.

Make a dressing with ¼ cup salad oil, 1 tablespoon lemon juice and 1 tablespoon cognac. Pour the dressing over the orange slices and chill well before serving. This salad should be garnished with a few sprigs of watercress.

• *Blender Gazpacho—Suzy Parker*

> *1 cup skinned, seeded cucumbers*
> *3 cups skinned, seeded tomatoes*
> *1 cup beef consommé*
> *4 teaspoons to 2 tablespoons salad oil*
> *1 teaspoon salt*
> *2 tablespoons chopped onion*
> *2 tablespoons chopped green pepper*
> *4 cloves garlic, chopped*

Blend together for 1 minute the cucumbers, tomatoes and consommé. Add the rest of the ingredients and blend for a few seconds more. Correct seasoning. Chill. Serve ice cold. Serves 4 or 5.

• *Boiled Artichokes Vinaigrette—Heather Bernard*

> *Cook 4 artichokes until tender. Cool.*
> *Make a vinaigrette sauce as follows:*
> *1 chopped hard-cooked egg*
> *1 tablespoon chopped chives*
> *1 tablespoon chopped parsley*
> *2 tablespoons chopped scallions or onions*
> *2 tablespoons chopped sweet pepper*
> *1 cup salad oil*
> *2 tablespoons lemon juice*
> *1 tablespoon English mustard*
> *1 tablespoon water*
> *1 teaspoon salt*

Mix all ingredients until blended well. Serve with artichokes.
Serves 4.

• Zucchini in a Pan alla Signora Piazzi

> 2 tablespoons bacon fat
> 1 medium onion, sliced
> 1 cup chopped tomatoes, canned or fresh
> ¾ teaspoon salt
> freshly ground black pepper to taste
> ½ bay leaf
> 3 medium zucchini, cut into 1-inch pieces

Heat the fat, add the onion and sauté until transparent. Add the tomatoes, salt, pepper and bay leaf. Simmer 5 minutes. Add the zucchini to the sauce, cover and simmer until tender, about 8 to 10 minutes.

• Red Cabbage with Apples—Trice Tomsen

> 1 medium head of red cabbage
> 2 tablespoons vinegar
> 2 onions
> 3 tablespoons margarine
> 3 tablespoons bacon fat
> 1 cup red wine
> 6 tart apples, peeled and sliced
> 1 bay leaf
> 4 cloves
> 2 peppercorns
> juice of ½ lemon, or to taste
> salt

Remove coarse or wilted outside leaves but do not wash the cabbage; slice very fine. Stuff it all into a glass jar; add the vinegar, stir, and leave for 20 minutes. Chop up the onions and brown them slowly in a saucepan, using 2 tablespoons margarine and all the bacon fat. When the onions are brown, put them, with as much of the cabbage as can be held comfortably at first, into a casserole or saucepan. Cook for a few minutes, turning and stirring the cabbage; then add more cabbage as the first cabbage becomes limp with cooking. When all cabbage has been put into the pot and has become limp, add the wine. Turn and stir carefully and add the apples, the bay leaf, cloves, peppercorns and a little salt. Cover loosely and cook over very low heat for about 30 minutes, or until the cabbage and the apples are tender and the moisture is absorbed. Stir from time to time; add lemon juice and salt to taste. Just before serving add the remaining tablespoon of margarine. Serves 4.

DAY 9

MENU

Breakfast

1,000 units vitamin C
1 multipurpose vitamin pill that contains minerals
1 cup of freshly squeezed grapefruit juice combined with
⅓ cup of Gevral protein supplement.

Lunch

Watercress and Endive Salad—Ann Turkel

Dinner

Eggplant Appetizer al Papacito Martin
Steamed Broccoli—Veronica Hamel
Spinach Rings with Carrots—Princess Grace of Monaco

• *Watercress and Endive Salad—Ann Turkel*

2 bunches watercress, washed and dried, stems removed
2 heads Belgian endive, chopped

Combine above ingredients in a salad bowl. Make the following dressing:

> ½ cup salad oil
> 2 teaspoons salt
> 2 tablespoons lemon juice
> 2 tablespoons tarragon vinegar
> 2 tablespoons chopped chives
> 2 tablespoons water
> 1 tablespoon freshly ground pepper

Combine ingredients in a deep bowl and beat with a whisk. Pour over the salad and mix well. Serves 4 generously.

• *Eggplant Appetizer al Papacito Martin*

> 2 medium eggplants
> 1 teaspoon lemon juice
> 1 teaspoon minced onion
> 1 cup diced celery
> ¼ cup French dressing
> Romaine or Bibb lettuce
> Garnish: quartered hard-boiled eggs, olives

Peel and cube eggplant. Cook in salted water with lemon juice. When eggplant is tender, drain and cool. Mix with onion, celery and French dressing. Chill. Serve on Romaine or Bibb lettuce. Garnish with quartered hard-boiled eggs and olives. Serves 4–6.

• *Steamed Broccoli—Veronica Hamel*

> 1 medium head of broccoli
> ½ stick margarine, melted

Steam broccoli in vegetable or clam steamer until just tender. Do not overcook. Serve with melted margarine poured over it.

• *Spinach Rings with Carrots—Princess Grace of Monaco*

> *2 pounds fresh spinach*
> *salt and freshly ground black pepper*
> *⅛ teaspoon nutmeg*
> *¼ cup margarine*
> *⅔ bunch carrots*
> *1½ cups chopped parsley*

Cook the spinach in the least possible water, drain and chop. Press all the moisture from the spinach before measuring. There should be 2 cups. Season with salt, pepper and nutmeg. Melt half the margarine and stir into the spinach. Pack into a well-margarined ring mold. Bake in a medium oven for 20 minutes. Keep hot until serving time. Scrape and trim the carrots and cut them lengthwise into thin strips about 1½ inches long. Cook them in salted water to cover until tender, about 6 to 8 minutes. Drain them, add the remaining margarine and the parsley, and toss to mix well. Unmold the spinach ring and fill the center with the buttered carrots. Serves 4.

DAY 10

MENU

Breakfast

> 1,000 units vitamin C
> 1 multipurpose vitamin pill that contains minerals
> 1 cup of freshly squeezed grapefruit juice combined with
> ⅓ cup of Gevral protein supplement.

Lunch

> Champignons à la Grecque—April and Jo

Dinner

> Cold Asparagus Vinaigrette—Corinne Spier
> Broiled Stuffed Mushrooms—Bjorn Axen
> Mashed Winter Squash—Mikael Katz
> Fried Cabbage—Loretta Otte

• *Champignons à la Grecque—April & Jo*

> *Bring to a boil the following mixture:*
> *½ cup water*
> *juice of half a lemon*
> *3 ounces salad oil*
> *sprig of thyme*
> *1 bay leaf and 1 stalk celery, tied together*
> *ground black pepper*
> *salt*
> *20 coriander seeds*
> *½ pound small white mushrooms, rubbed clean with a*
> *paper towel, not peeled*

Boil all ingredients except the mushrooms for 10 minutes. Lower heat and simmer 5 minutes more. Drain. Let mushrooms rest in marinade for several hours. Serve cold with a little of the marinade on lettuce leaves. Serves 2.

• *Cold Asparagus Vinaigrette—Corinne Spier*

> *2 pounds asparagus*
> *⅓ cup red wine vinegar*
> *½ teaspoon sharp mustard*
> *1 clove garlic, minced*
> *¾ teaspoon salt*
> *⅛ teaspoon pepper*
> *⅔ cup salad oil*
> *1 small can red pimentos*
> *3 tablespoons chopped parsley*

Wash and trim the asparagus. Place on a trivet in boiling salted water in a deep frying pan (or stand upright in bottom of a double boiler with top section inverted as a cover). Boil 10 to 12 minutes. Drain thoroughly and chill in the refrigerator. Combine the remaining ingredients (except the pimentos and parsley) for the dressing. Chill. Cut the pimentos into thin strips. Arrange the cold asparagus on individual plates. Garnish each serving with the strips of pimento and a sprinkling of parsley. Spoon a little of the well-mixed dressing on each portion of asparagus and serve the rest in a separate bowl. Serves 4.

• Broiled Stuffed Mushrooms—Bjorn Axen

Preheat broiler. Remove stems and wipe with a damp cloth 12 large mushroom caps. Chop the stems. Simmer them for 2 minutes in 1 tablespoon margarine.

Add 1½ tablespoons chopped chives and tarragon, mixed, and ½ cup chopped parsley.

Bind these ingredients with a little melted margarine. Season with salt and paprika. Brush the caps with butter or olive oil. Fill them with the above stuffing and sprinkle with grated Parmesan cheese. Place mushrooms cap side up on a well-greased pan. Broil for about 5 minutes and serve them sizzling hot. Serves 4.

• Mashed Winter Squash—Mikael Katz

Preheat oven to 375° F. Scrub: a 3- to 4-pound Hubbard or other winter squash. Place squash on a rack and bake it until it can be pierced easily with a toothpick. Cut it in halves and remove the seeds. Peel the squash and mash the pulp. To each cup of squash add 1 tablespoon margarine, ¼ teaspoon salt, ⅛ teaspoon ginger. Beat this well with enough orange juice to make it of good consistency. Place mixture in a bake-and-serve casserole and reheat in medium oven. Sprinkle with ¼ cup crushed pineapple. Serves 6.

• *Fried Cabbage—Loretta Otte*

> *1 small head of cabbage*
> *6 tablespoons melted bacon fat or, if not available, margarine*

Parboil cabbage in boiling salted water for 5 minutes. Remove from water and slice fine. Sauté until cabbage is well coated with hot bacon fat or margarine that has been browned in a skillet. Serves 3 or 4.

DAY 11

MENU

Breakfast

> 1,000 units vitamin C
> 1 multipurpose vitamin pill that contains minerals
> 1 cup of freshly squeezed grapefruit juice combined with ⅓ cup of Gevral protein supplement

Lunch

> Jamie Craft's Salad

Dinner

> Spinach à la Jennifer O'Neill
> Eggplant Soufflé—Darling Charles
> Stewed Tomatoes—Kay Bourland

• Jamie Craft's Salad

Combine equal parts of sliced, unpeeled cucumber (if unwaxed—otherwise peel them) cooked asparagus tips, cooked green beans cut in ½-inch lengths, and small, raw cauliflower flowerets. Mix with mayonnaise to which a little yogurt and a few pinches of dried chervil and tarragon have been added. Heap into a mound and serve on shredded lettuce mixed with watercress leaves.

• Spinach à la Jennifer O'Neill

Wash well and remove the coarse stems from 1 pound spinach. Shake off as much water as possible. Heat in a large, heavy skillet 1 tablespoon margarine and 2 tablespoons salad oil. Add 1 clove minced garlic. Add the spinach. Cover at once and cook over high heat until steam appears. Reduce the heat and simmer until tender, 5 to 6 minutes in all. Stir in 2 tablespoons pignolis (pine nuts). Serve hot. Serves 2 or 3.

• Eggplant Soufflé—Darling Charles

> 1 medium-size eggplant
> ¾ cup sautéed onions
> 2 beaten egg yolks
> 1 tablespoon melted margarine
> ½ cup chopped skim-milk mozzarella
> salt and pepper
> grated nutmeg
> 2 egg whites

Preheat oven to 325° F. Parboil eggplant for 10 minutes. Slice it in half, scooping out the pulp. Keep shells intact. Mash the pulp. Combine it with the onions, egg yolks, margarine, mozzarella and seasonings. Mix well. Beat egg whites until stiff but not dry. Fold them lightly into eggplant mixture. Fill the shells. Place them in a baking pan with a little water and bake for about 30 minutes. Serves 2.

• Stewed Tomatoes—Kay Bourland

> 6 large tomatoes (or 2½ cups canned tomatoes)
> 1 teaspoon minced onion
> 1½ cups chopped celery
> 2 or 3 cloves
> 1 tablespoon margarine
> ¾ teaspoon salt
> ¼ teaspoon paprika
> ⅛ teaspoon curry powder
> 1 teaspoon chopped parsley

If using fresh tomatoes, wash and skin them and cut into quarters. Place them in a heavy pan over low heat and cook for about 20 minutes. If using canned tomatoes, heat through and let simmer for 10 minutes. Add the onion, celery and cloves while tomatoes are cooking or heating through. Stir occasionally to keep from scorching. Before serving add the margarine, salt, paprika, curry powder and parsley. Serves 4 or 5.

DAY 12

MENU

Breakfast

1,000 units vitamin C
1 multipurpose vitamin pill that contains minerals
1 cup of freshly squeezed grapefruit juice combined with
⅓ cup of Gevral protein supplement

Lunch

Lettuce with Melted Margarine—Katie Scarlett

Dinner

> Sliced Tomatoes with Anchovy and Beet Dressing—
> G.W.F., Jr.
> Zucchini in Dill—Bo Appeltoft
> Steamed Asparagus—Lacey Ford

• *Lettuce with Melted Margarine—Katie Scarlett*

Use only the tenderest of lettuce hearts for this exquisite salad. Arrange them in a salad bowl, season them very lightly with salt and a pinch of sugar, and at the last moment pour over them warm melted margarine into which you have pounded a small piece of garlic and a squeeze of lemon juice.

• *Sliced Tomatoes with Anchovy and Beet Dressing— G.W.F. Jr.*

> *Place in a jar with a screw top:*
> *½ cup French dressing (salad oil and vinegar, half and half)*
> *2 tablespoons water*
> *3 or 4 anchovies, chopped*
> *2 small cooked beets, chopped*
> *1 hard-boiled egg, chopped*
> *salt and pepper to taste (dressing should be spicy)*
> *firm ripe tomatoes in quantity desired*

Put all ingredients except tomatoes into jar and shake jar well until dressing is thoroughly blended. Pour the dressing over sliced tomatoes just before serving.

• Zucchini in Dill—Bo Appeltoft

> *4 small raw zucchini, washed and sliced about ⅛ inch thick*
> *1 teaspoon salt*
> *1 tablespoon Colman's mustard*
> *½ cup salad oil*
> *2 tablespoons cold water*
> *4 tablespoons lemon juice*
> *4 tablespoons chopped fresh dill or 1 tablespoon dried dill*
> *4 tablespoons chopped raw onion*

Combine salt, mustard and oil with water. Beat with a whisk. Beat in lemon juice, stir in chopped dill and onion. Pour over raw zucchini and serve on a bed of Romaine or other lettuce leaves. Serves 4.

• Steamed Asparagus with Melted Margarine—Lacey Ford

> *1 bunch asparagus*
> *1 stick margarine, melted*

Trim asparagus and tie together. Cook standing up until barely tender in an asparagus steamer, or in the bottom of a double boiler with top reversed for a cover so that it will serve as a steamer. Serve with melted margarine poured over. Serves 3 or 4.

DAY 13

MENU

Breakfast

> 1,000 units vitamin C
> 1 multipurpose vitamin pill that contains minerals
> 1 cup of freshly squeezed grapefruit juice combined with
> ⅓ cup of Gevral protein supplement

Lunch

> Tomato, Mozzarella and Basil Salad—Parco dei Principi

Dinner

> Sautéed Eggplant Slices—Riccardo Gay
> Grilled Tomatoes—Ewa Karrlander
> Steamed Broccoli with Blender Hollandaise—George
> Hamilton

• *Tomato, Mozzarella and Basil Salad—Parco dei Principi*

Slice several large ripe tomatoes. Top these with thick slices of skim-milk mozzarella. Add cut-up leaves of fresh basil or sprinkle with dried basil—or if you prefer, add basil to salad dressing. Cover with homemade French dressing (any you prefer).

• *Sautéed Eggplant Slices—Riccardo Gay*

Peel and cut into ½ inch slices, cubes or sticks, 1 eggplant. Dip the pieces in milk. Dust them with a little flour. For easier handling, place slices on a rack to dry for 15 minutes before cooking. Melt a little butter or oil in a skillet. Sauté the pieces until tender. Serve while hot with chopped parsley or tarragon, lemon slices or tomato sauce. Serves 3 or 4.

• Grilled Tomatoes—Ewa Karrlander

Preheat broiler. Wash 4 large, firm tomatoes. Cut them crosswise into even ½-inch slices. Season them well with 1 teaspoon salt, ¼ teaspoon pepper and a pinch of celery salt. Place in a greased pan and cover them with 1 cup sour cream mixed with 2 tablespoons of grated onion. Broil them for about 10 minutes, about 5 inches below the broiler flame.

• Steamed Broccoli with Blender Hollandaise—
George Hamilton

> 1 bunch broccoli
> 3 egg yolks
> 2 tablespoons lemon juice
> pinch of cayenne
> ¼ teaspoon salt
> 1 cup margarine

Wash the broccoli and steam until barely tender. In the meantime, place in the blender the egg yolks, the lemon juice, the cayenne and salt. Heat the margarine to bubbling, but do not brown. Cover blender container and turn motor to "high." After 3 seconds, remove the lid and pour the margarine over the egg mixture in a steady stream. By the time all the margarine is poured in—about 30 seconds—the sauce should be finished. If not, blend, still on "high" about 5 seconds longer. Serve at once over the broccoli—or keep sauce warm by immersing container in warm water. Serves 4.

Note: Do not make hollandaise in a smaller quantity than given here.

DAY 14

MENU

Breakfast

> 1,000 units vitamin C
> 1 multipurpose vitamin pill that contains minerals
> 1 cup of freshly squeezed grapefruit juice combined with
> ⅓ cup of Gevral protein supplement

Lunch

> Tomatoes with Cucumber Ice—Inger Malmeroos

Dinner

> Mushroom Salad—Birte Strandgaard
> Mixed Vegetable Grill—Sunny Griffin
> Italian Spinach—Soni C.

• *Tomatoes with Cucumber Ice—Inger Malmeroos*

Choose ripe, full-flavored tomatoes and do not peel the cucumber unless the skin has been waxed.

> *2 or 3 cucumbers*
> *3 tablespoons white wine vinegar*
> *1 teaspoon salt*
> *¼ teaspoon pepper*
> *½ envelope unflavored gelatin*
> *3 tablespoons cold water*
> *6 medium-size ripe tomatoes*
> *lettuce*

Quarter cucumbers lengthwise, remove seeds and grate or chop fine in an electric blender (there should be about 2 cups, including juice). Add vinegar, salt and pepper. Soften gelatin in cold water and dissolve over hot water. Add to cucumber, turn into freezing tray and freeze until almost firm. Transfer to chilled bowl, beat well and return to tray. Freeze again. Slice tomatoes downward into 6 or 8 sections, leaving them attached at the base. Place each on a lettuce leaf and put a scoop of cucumber ice in the center of each one. Serves 5 or 6.

• Mushroom Salad—Birte Strandgaard

1 tablespoon salt
4 teaspoons dry mustard
½ cup salad oil
2 tablespoons water
4 tablespoons lemon juice
a few grinds of black pepper
2 tablespoons sour cream
½ pound raw mushrooms, wiped clean and sliced thin
   (if stems are firm and white, they may be included)

Combine salt, mustard and oil with water. Beat in lemon juice and pepper with a whisk. Stir in sour cream. Mix well with raw mushrooms. Serve on lettuce leaves. Serves 2 or 3.

• Mixed Vegetable Grill—Sunny Griffin

Preheat broiler. Cut into thick slices firm, ripe tomatoes in quantity desired. Brush with melted margarine and season with salt, pepper and a little basil (fresh or dried). Wipe clean as many mushrooms as desired. Brush with melted margarine and season with salt and pepper. Grease broiler and arrange on it the tomato slices and the mushrooms. Broil until lightly browned. Serve at once on a platter garnished with parsley, olives, radishes or other herbs and vegetables as you wish.

• *Italian Spinach—Soni C.*

> *2 pounds spinach, well washed and trimmed*
> *3 tablespoons margarine*
> *4 tablespoons salad oil*
> *1 clove garlic, finely chopped*
> *salt to taste*
> *¼ teaspoon cayenne pepper*
> *coarsely grated Parmesan cheese*

Cut the spinach into coarse shreds. Drop into small amount of boiling salted water and cook for 30 seconds. Drain well, pressing out excess moisture, and place in a baking dish. In a skillet, heat the margarine and oil. Add the garlic, salt and cayenne, and cook over low heat 5 minutes. Combine the oil mixture with the spinach in the baking dish and sprinkle with cheese and additional margarine, melted. Brown quickly under a broiler. Serves 4 or 5.

The diet is really scrumptious; but if it is to be fully effective, some exercises should go along with it.

I've come up with fourteen exercises, each to be done for one minute each day. These will, if done religiously, really snap you into shape in fourteen days. They are not easy, however, and should be done sensibly; don't exceed your capabilities. You'll get there in time.

I take a copy of the exercises wherever I go, and the only problem I've encountered are the shrieks of the poor people who have the room under mine when I do the jogging exercise. It's hard to jog quietly even on tiptoe.

You have only one body in your lifetime, and you might as

well take the best possible care of it that you can. Later on in these pages, I'll tell you how to maintain your new weight and figure.

1. Jog in place for one minute.

2. Stand with legs astride. Clasp hands overhead. Bend sideways to the right and bounce twice to the right, return to upright position and bounce twice to the left. Do this exercise rapidly, inhaling and exhaling as you do. Repeat for one minute.

3. Clasp hands on head with palms facing upwards. Inhale as you slowly push your palms and arms upward as if you were pushing a weight. Push until you can feel a good stretch in your lower abdomen and waist. Lower hands to head slowly, exhaling as you do. Repeat for one minute.

4. Stand with feet wide apart, toes pointing outward. Bend forward at hip joints and place hands on knees. Shift your weight to the right, bending your right knee and straightening your left leg as you do. Then shift weight to left side with left knee bent and right leg straight. Try to get a nice flowing rhythm as you shift weight from one side to the other. Repeat for one minute.

5. Hold onto back of chair or to table. Pull in buttocks, buttock muscles pushing forward as you do. Tighten abdomen muscles at same time. Still keeping these muscles tight, stretch right leg back at an angle to your body. Pointing your toes, bring leg up, then down, toes touching the floor at the down thrust. Do this for 30 seconds. Repeat, this time with the left leg, for 30 seconds more. It is essential that you keep the abdomen and buttock muscles tight throughout the exercise.

6. Sit on floor with hands in back touching floor for support. Extend legs in front of you and lift them alternately, first right, then left. Repeat this swiftly for one minute.

7. Stand with right leg extended forward, left leg extended to the rear. Extend left arm forward, right arm back. Jump in place and reverse this position, left leg and right arm forward, right leg and left arm to the rear. Repeat swiftly, alternating arms and legs and inhaling and exhaling as you do. Repeat for one minute.

8. Jog in place as if to the beat of a tom-tom for one minute.

9. Sit on floor with hands behind you on floor for support. Bend knees and place feet flat on floor. With feet, knees and legs together, pull up toward right shoulder, return feet to floor and pull up toward left shoulder, always keeping feet, knees and legs together. Repeat, alternating from right side to left, for one minute. You should get a good twist at the waist as you do this exercise.

10. Stand with feet slightly apart. Cross arms and place hands on opposite shoulders, inhaling as you do. Slowly bend forward at the waist, allowing arms and hands to fall limply toward floor. Exhale while bending forward. Cross arms again and slowly straighten up, tightening all muscles including calves, thighs, buttocks and abdomen. Inhale as you return to upright position. Repeat for one minute.

11. Sit on floor, reclining on elbows. Bend knees and place feet flat on floor about eighteen inches from buttocks. Raise feet and legs so that calves form right angle to floor. From this position raise and then lower legs and feet to floor. Repeat for one minute.

12. Lie on back. Raise legs at right angles to body, straight in the air, toes pointed toward the ceiling. Slowly open and close legs in scissors motion tightening inner thigh muscles as you close legs. If you wish, you can do this exercise by gradually lowering legs to floor as you do scissors, but it's difficult. Repeat for one minute.

13. Kneel on floor, sitting on heels. Extend arms at shoulder level straight in front of you. Raise your body to erect kneeling position, pulling up with abdomen muscles; inhale as you do. Return to

sitting-on-heels position, trying to keep muscles tightened, and exhale as you do. Repeat for one minute.

14. Jog in place for one minute.

3

Sex and What to Do About It

There are an awesome number of books about sex on the market, and many of them turn into best-sellers. Why? Because all of us are searching for a way to perfect, or maybe just reinforce, our relationship with the man in our lives.

It would be difficult in these times for all of us not to realize what's going on around us. Men are leaving their wives right and left for younger women. I really and sincerely believe that all too often the wife is at fault. Not only has she let herself go physically; she has forgotten the importance of an active and exciting sex life.

Taking care of a home and children or going to business or both can consume so much of a woman's time and energies that she will all too often forget about, or feel too tired for, sex. You just can't do that. Children and homes and careers are great. Ask me—I've had all three, and they're all in their own ways marvelous and nothing would or could replace them in my life. But sex—well, I've tried that too and it's great, and nothing, I repeat, *nothing*, will ever replace it as the vital force in any relationship between a man and woman. It is indeed the tie that binds.

Am I saying that sex is the most important facet in keeping people together? Yes, I am. Of course there has to be love and tenderness; there are myriad other facets to keeping people together in a happy state of being. However, an active, mutually responsive sex life is the cornerstone of that relationship.

Sex, to a man, is an affirmation of his masculinity. If you take this away from a man, if you fail to reaffirm his masculinity, then you take away a good part of his ego—so necessary to his self-esteem. I realize that this concept may seem outmoded in a world where women are constantly being told that they should be "equal." There are many ways in which a woman can assert her equality: equal pay for equal work, freedom to choose her role in life. If that's what you want, fine, be equal; however I sincerely believe that if you want to be cherished and loved over any great length of time, you can't imitate men. Leave masculinity to them and be a complete woman yourself. When men are more masculine, women become more feminine. I've had many opportunities to see many different ways of living, and from what I've seen, the woman who is feminine has a much better life.

Women think they need constant reassurance that they are loved, wanted and cherished. Men need it too; their egos are even more fragile than ours! A man can't come out and ask for emotional reassurance the way a woman can. That is one reason men need this reassurance even more than women do. A good home, a loving woman who looks her best, are all well and good as indications of love, but a sexually responsive woman is the most important indicator of all.

I don't mean a body that is available on demand; when I say "responsive" I mean just that—an enthusiastic, creative partner is all-important to a man. Men need satisfying sexual relationships. Sex to a man is a much more direct affirmation of love than it is to a woman. A man seems to feel that sex expresses emotions that women can feel more easily than they: affection, reassurance, tenderness. A man may not even feel free to admit to himself or to his partner that he is looking for those emotions. If he isn't receiving all this from you he may believe that he can receive it from some other woman who is either more responsive or is capable of putting on a good act. She may be your age or a younger woman who hasn't yet settled down and become involved in day-to-day living. The "who" doesn't matter. All she has to be is there and giving—not just taking.

Most married men are just not looking for a new woman. Men who are are largely driven to it by their wives, who have neglected this side of marriage. Men don't really want a new body; they want the girl they once knew and loved enough to marry. If they are looking for new partners, it is because they are seeking that same enthusiastic response their wives once gave them. I'm not saying that sex in itself is the only thing of importance to a man. Sex is important, yes—but only with all those other components of love and tenderness does it become all-important.

All the books and articles that tell women how to attract lovers stress one thing over and over and over again. A man needs a responsive, enthusiastic, alluring partner. A wife of many years often ignores this counsel—it comes to younger women naturally. A young wife makes a man believe he can relive his youth, when he knew he was wanted and loved and welcomed in bed—not as an obligation, but with real responsiveness and a will to be an active participant.

Are you at this point about to ask if this need doesn't grow less with the mature years? Doesn't all the richness of a shared life, or so many years together, more than take the place of plain old sex?

Not at all! Nothing takes the place of sex at any time. The need for sex is lifelong. As long as you want to keep the man in your life interested in you, as long as you yourself want to keep vibrantly alive, as long as you want to enjoy the fullness of living, that's just how long you will need and want sex.

Sex goes on for the length of your life. Sex is a giving of love, a sharing of love. When you lose your interest in sex, you are telling your husband you are no longer as interested in him as you were at the beginning of your marriage. Without putting it into words, you are saying that he doesn't have enough to offer you to keep your interest alive. This is the death blow to the male ego.

Can you blame the man who wants to heal this wound in any way he can when you tell him, in effect, that he can't convey love and pleasure to you, that he's not really the man he thinks he is? Can you find it in your heart to be angry with him for looking elsewhere for reassurance? The need for love and affection can motivate a man in any direction. That direction is up to you.

Suppose you are one of those who are genuinely, really and truly, too tired at the end of a day to enjoy lovemaking. That is a problem you must solve. There are health-and-energy-giving exercises that will guarantee you that young-woman feeling! If you need them, you'll find them right here in this chapter.

Some women face a subtler problem in the sharing of sexual relations. I know that there are many wives who want to continue the pleasure of an active sex life but who don't know how to convey this feeling to their husbands. This can be devastating. Some women think, often unconsciously, that only the male is allowed to make overt sexual advances; that women can flirt and lead on and lure, but to indicate outright sexual desire—no. But there are times, lots of times, when men love to have the woman play the role of the sexual aggressor. It's true. A man may be tired, or simply in a passive mood, yet desire sexual relations perhaps even more than at other times, simply because he needs the comfort more. You know how flattered you feel when a man indicates that you are desirable. A man has exactly the same feeling—even more so. A little aggression on your part can serve you in good stead, not just once; it can start you on the road to being lovers again. We went to Capri on a vacation and Jerry fell into the Italian habit of a siesta. One day I just woke him up by several sexy gestures, and believe me, it started a whole new and even more delightful sexual relationship. I don't know why my aggression triggered it; I can just tell you it did.

But you may have been, consciously or not, sending out rejection signals. You may have felt that it's somehow undignified for a settled couple still to have a passionate interest in sex. I don't know why! It's healthful for you and your husband, and it can be fun! You may, as I've indicated, really be tired; you may want sex but you wish it weren't so boring, cut-and-dried, the same old thing. You just may not know how to get it going.

Whatever the reason, do something about it. If the spark is gone from your sex life, you've had it. Sooner or later you'll be in bed alone. Your husband isn't going to make love to you if he thinks he's going to be rebuffed or unsatisfied. A marriage without satisfactory, joyous, delicious sex is a marriage that isn't going to last. It isn't death that will you part; you can count on that.

You must forget the old saw that sex is only for the young. It's amazing how these old beliefs cling to us—you might as well say that eating is only for the young. We all need food to keep our bodies alive. We all need sex to keep our vitality alive. I can't repeat this too often: *There is no end to the desire for sex.* There is no reason that it should ever end. The act of love is satisfying at all ages when it is performed with love and obvious enjoyment.

The above paragraph should go into your subconscious. Carry it around with you. No matter what your age, you are alive, you love, you are worthy of love and being loved. Sex is the natural form of love. So express that love naturally and with gusto!

There is nothing in the way of lovemaking that is illicit between two people who love each other. There are plenty of good books about sex on the market. Read them if you need them. And then follow them. If you're clumsy at first, do the exercises in this chapter to improve your mobility; practice makes perfect. As one airline used to say, "Getting there is half the fun."

The first step in revitalizing your sex life is thinking, feeling, acting sensuously. The next step in convincing your husband

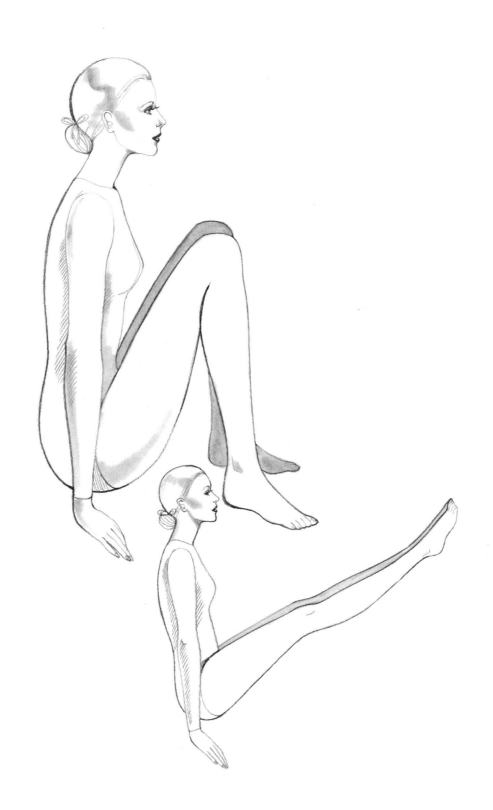

that you are eager for his lovemaking is a body toned, alive, responsive. Here are the exercises that will most effectively help you to your goal. They limber and develop the right muscles to make you active in your sex life. It may take time to develop them, but once you do, your sex life can be as active as anyone's—maybe even more so. Use these muscles as you develop. Practice really can make you perfect!

PELVIC FLEXIBILITY EXERCISE: Get down on all fours, keeping the elbows straight. Now, in the way a cat arches its spine— slowly, easily—arch your spine. Then let it come down slowly into a concave position, keeping your elbows straight. *Don't hurry.* Do this three times. Then rest. This exercise increases the flexibility of the whole pelvic area. Incidentally, it is one of the best pre- and post-natal exercises going.

ABDOMEN-STRENGTHENING EXERCISE: Sit on the floor with your feet out in front of you. Rest your palms on the floor, one on each side of you. Inhale slowly. Draw your knees up. Now straighten out your legs, and keep them straight, as you raise the legs only, as close to an angle of 45 degrees as you can get. Lean back slightly, pressing your palms to the floor to balance yourself. Hold for only a few seconds, then exhale and bring your legs down. Your abdomen will be greatly strengthened as well as flattened.

What comes next is a specific exercise to train the vaginal muscles. It's simple and basic, and while it is useful in itself, it can be employed in conjunction with some other exercises I am going to give you later.

Right now, as you are sitting, see if you can't press the labia and sphincter muscles together. (These are the opening and inner passage.) The easiest way to get these internal muscles working for you is to pretend that you need to urinate but can't get to the bathroom quickly enough. You will automatically tighten the correct muscles. Now release. This is an isometric exercise. Just a few times a day, whenever you think of it, do this vaginal tightening-and-releasing routine. Tightening and releasing during lovemaking adds immeasurably to a man's pleasure.

Here is a group of exercises designed specifically to make you more limber when you make love. It goes without saying that a woman who participates fully, who is able to be very active, not only gives but receives more pleasure than a woman who is passive and stiff. It never hurts to practice keeping your body supple and limber.

The Basic Exercise: Lie flat on your stomach, comfortably. Fold your elbows and let your head rest on them. Draw in the muscles of your buttocks against each other. Hold; then relax. Do this a few times. Then, at the same time, try to pull in the abdomen as you tighten your buttocks. After you can do the two with ease simultaneously, add the inner tightening that we mentioned before. When you can do all three simultaneously, tightening and relaxing without any great effort, do the exercise quickly—but always easily. Ten times a day is a good number, do more if you feel like it.

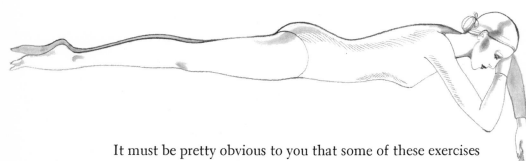

It must be pretty obvious to you that some of these exercises you are doing on the exercise floor are what you should be doing in bed. Your abdomen should be firm, hard, toned, so that you can not only support the weight of your husband but can move your entire body easily during the sex act. Your vaginal muscles should be firm, yet limber, so that they will be a supporting yet caressing sheath for your husband. It is much more pleasurable for both of you when you can control that complicated stretch of muscles inside the vaginal passage during lovemaking. For instance, at times when he is tired, your alternate loosening and tightening of the vagina will give him maximum pleasure with much less effort on his part. If this sounds like reversing the roles, if you are active and he is passive, that is part of the give and take of lovemaking.

HIP SUPPLENESS EXERCISE: This one is simple. Take a stance with feet wide apart. Keeping the knees stiff, swing the hips to the right as far as possible. Without twisting the body,

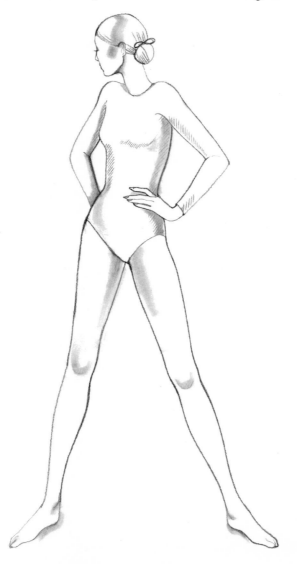

swing to the left. Keep the knees stiff and shoulders straight and level. Everything in between should be taut. Since you already know how to pull in the abdomen and buttocks, this shouldn't be at all difficult. A few swings like this a day will make you most flexible in love.

ALL-OVER EXERCISES: If you ever have seen genuine Oriental dancing, you will have seen how supple the muscles used in making love can be. What you don't see is the effect some of these movements can have on the interior muscles. They do indeed—and you can certainly learn them for yourself. It sounds a little complicated at first, but with practice it all becomes surprisingly easy. Do the following exercises smoothly, please; don't force anything, or you will lose all the benefit.

Stand with your feet slightly apart, about six inches, and your knees relaxed. *One:* Tilt your pelvis forward. Tighten your inner vaginal muscles. *Two:* Put your weight on your right foot and thrust your hips to the right side; relax the vaginal muscles when you do this. *Three:* Tilt your pelvis back and tighten your vaginal muscles. *Four:* Shift the hips to the left, weight on the left foot, and relax the vaginal muscles. Do this set of four movements, always starting with the hips shifted to the right, four times. Keep careful count. Now reverse, doing four sets, starting with the left foot and left hip. It's important that you relax and tighten the vaginal muscles on the proper movement.

When you have gotten this series of movements down so that you can easily shift, tighten, relax (it should only take you a few days) then you turn the whole thing into the dance movement. You do the same movements in a circle. Feet slightly apart, knees thoroughly relaxed, tilt pelvis forward, right, back, left forward, all in one smooth motion. Meanwhile, you will be tightening and relaxing your interior muscles automatically, as you will be doing from now on when you make love.

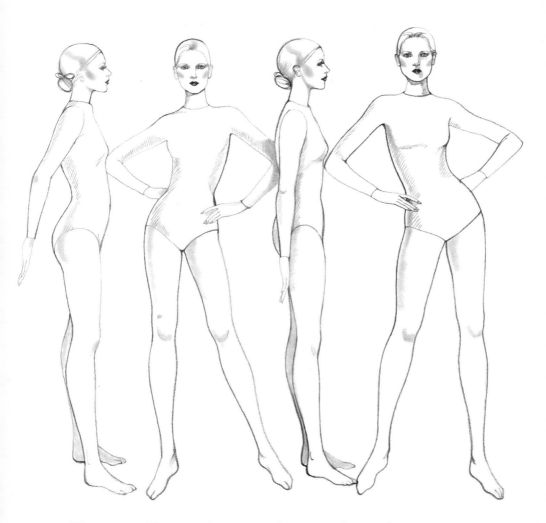

VARIATION: You may have seen that same dancer do a provocative movement: she puts her hands on her knees and wiggles. Here is the basis of it.

Stand with your feet apart, your knees bent. Place your hands on your knees, push your buttocks out behind you and arch your back as much as you comfortably can. Now straighten out, pulling in all interior and exterior muscles, but keep your hands on your knees. Your back will arch outward a little; the rest of you will pull in. This exercise, incidentally, is wonderful for flattening the abdomen. Hold this position for

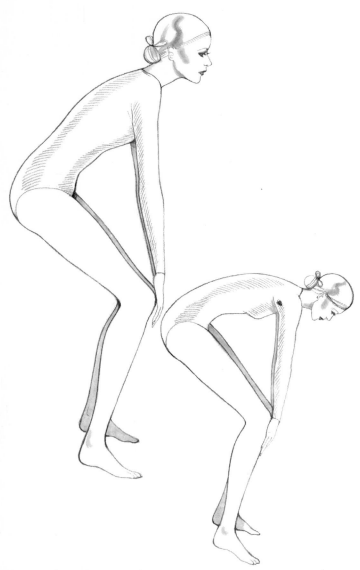

a slow count of three to five; then repeat three to five times.
When you become adept, as you will in a short time, you will
be able to do it as smoothly as the dancer does, and you might
want to try doing these movements in a slow circle as she does.
Do the exercise to music if possible.

For suppleness in the pelvic area, as well as limbering up the
spine (most important for enjoyable sex) try this one.

FORWARD STRETCH: Sit with your legs as far apart as is comfortable. Inhale. Then exhale and lean forward. Place your fingers on your toes and without bending the knees, try to bring your head to the floor. Do these movements gradually; don't force anything. As you grow more supple, the exercise will be easier and the effectiveness greater.

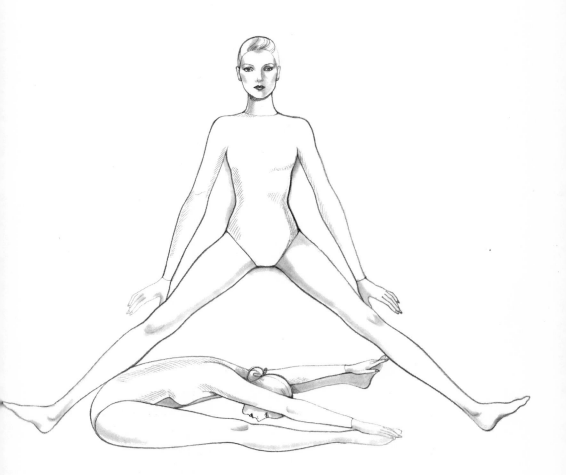

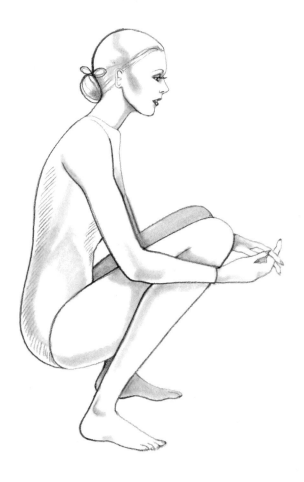

PELVIC TONE-UP: This is based on a yoga exercise. If you can sit back on your heels comfortably, do so. Otherwise sit with your legs crossed. Inhale. Exhale, drawing in the vaginal muscles. Try to draw them inward and upward. Hold for a moment, then relax. Again inhale, and while exhaling, contract. You can repeat this as often as you like, or as often as is comfortable. This exercise not only tones up the vaginal muscles, but is supposed to benefit a prolapsed uterus.

ALL-FOURS SWING: Get down on hands and knees. Swing the pelvis to the right and to the left, and as you repeat the movements, try to speed them up. Make sure all movements are from the waist down only. The rest of your body should be stationary.

VARIATION: In the same position, rotate the pelvis.

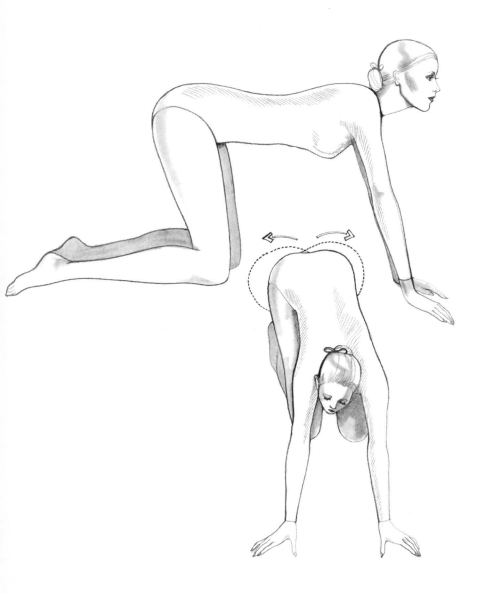

Leg Exercise: Lie on your back with your knees bent and your feet flat on the floor. Now try to separate your legs as if someone were holding them together. If you can't imagine the resistance, put your hands on your knees and try to pull them apart while at the same time your legs are resisting.

Any of these exercises should tone up the vaginal area, give you greater facility in sexual performance and help you to greater enjoyment in lovemaking than you have ever known. It's particularly important that you keep the vaginal muscles in good shape exactly as you would any other part of your body.

As you progress, you may want to try the following exercises, which are strictly intended to make you more active sexually. I am calling them "Pelvic Training Exercises" because that is exactly what they are.

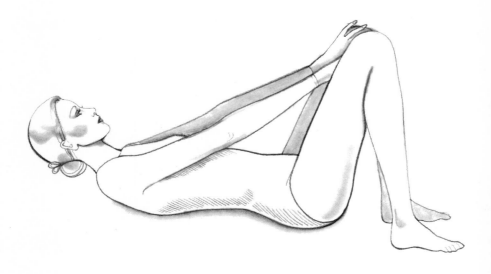

Basic: Lie flat on the floor, on a carpet or blanket. Place your feet about eighteen inches apart. Bring them up toward you so that your knees are bent. You should be comfortable. Keep your shoulders and buttocks on the floor and arch your back slightly. Then pull your spine flat down to the floor. While you are doing this, tighten your buttocks and the internal muscles. Hold for a count of three. Relax. Practice this till you can arch and relax ten times easily.

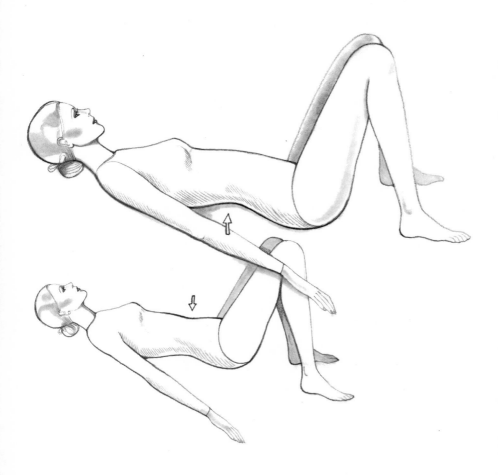

THIGH ACTION: Your thighs are important in lovemaking, as nobody need tell you. This exercise works on the pelvic area and the thighs, strengthening both. Get on your knees and sit on your heels. If you find that position painful for your ankles, roll up a small towel and let your ankles be supported by it. After a while you may be able to discard the towel.

At first you are sitting on your heels with your buttocks resting on them. Push your buttocks as far back as you can. Now, bring the buttocks under and the pelvis forward. Stretch your arms out in front of you to give you some balance, and try not to raise your head more than two or three inches. Return to the first position and relax. This is the same lovemaking move-

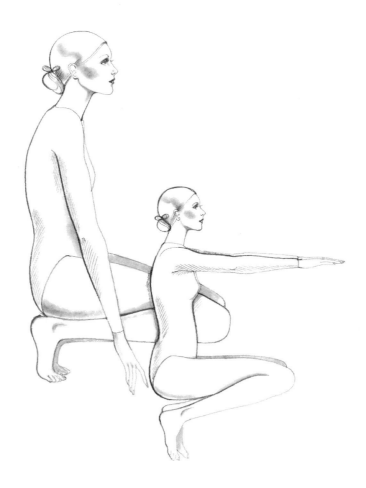

ment you have practiced on the floor, but with more effort involved and more strengthening results. You may not be able to do this more than once or twice a day for the first few days, but when your thighs develop strength and limberness, you may want to go up to eight times a day.

Flexibility is all-important in lovemaking. To keep your pelvic area flexible, try this simple exercise: Sit on the floor, your legs stretched before you. Now, without straining, place your feet with the soles touching each other. Your knees will be up from the floor. Now, grasping the ankles firmly, see how far you can press your knees to the floor. You won't be able to get them flat on the floor, so don't expect to. The idea is to see how far you can get them down without straining, which at the same time will flex the pelvic area. Don't hold the position longer than five seconds at a time. Work up to five stretches a day, always relaxing between stretches.

All or any of these exercises should do wonders for your sex life. Tone, limber and exercise, and you will make a wonderful bed partner.

Sometimes, however, a woman who has had several children or whose muscles for whatever reason have become too lapsed to benefit by exercise may want to try vaginal plastic surgery. Genital prolapse is correctable by surgery.

The muscles of the birth canal provide support to the pelvic organs, which include the rectum, bladder, uterus and vagina. During childbearing and delivery these muscles may be stretched. Among the various conditions that may result, the vaginal orifice may become so relaxed and weakened that it does not give the pleasure it once did in sexual relations.

These conditions can be improved or corrected with surgery. A gynecologist can tighten up the chain of muscles that make up the vaginal orifice. He can go back into what doctors call the vault, which is the upper part of the vagina, around the cervix, and tighten that area. Such correction of the torn or overstretched supporting structures and the vaginal wall and the muscles to the outlet of the vagina ought to do a great deal to bring back the pleasure in lovemaking that possibly you and your husband have missed lately.

There is also the problem of the vagina becoming dry as hormonal functions decrease, thus making intercourse painful. Your gynecologist can give you a hormonal cream to rectify this discomfort.

So there you are. If you have thought your sex life was over, think again. Dr. Mary Calderone, who ought to know, since she is one of the founders of SIECUS (Sex Information and Education Council of the United States) says that a woman's sex life goes on into her eighties. Beyond that, who knows? There is no reason to think that there is any age at which sex stops. What a lovely thought. An even lovelier thought is that you—that's right, little old you—can be practical and perfecting and really loving it every minute.

4

Eileen's Maintenance Diet

Before we go into the diet itself, let's consider the principles of good nourishment on which it was built—this new way of eating combines all the necessary nutrients you need to look and feel exciting as well as slender. You will notice that there is a great emphasis on *protein* foods. The word "protein," derived from the Greek, means "of first importance." Protein foods are the material of which living tissue is built. If there is not enough protein in your diet, muscles are likely to become flaccid. For instance, the so-called dowager's hump, which many women think is an inevitable accompaniment of old age, isn't inevitable at all. This hump is the slump of shoulder muscles that have been inadequately fed. Lack of protein may also show in the face, which is more apt to sag on a poor diet than on a good one. I don't care if you've read about food values before; read about them again. Knowing about them is essential to your better life plan.

The basic protein foods are: milk, meat, fowl, fish, cheese, eggs and yogurt.

Fats should never be eliminated entirely. For one thing, they are concentrated sources of energy. They also help to metabolize the fat-soluble vitamins, which are A, D, K and E. The proper fats are essential to the good health of the skin, and they help keep the hair in good condition. A moderate amount of fat should be taken every day in the form of natural vegetable oils: corn, cottonseed, safflower, peanut oils are all good. You will also find natural oils in fish and seafood.

Carbohydrates are another valuable form of nutrient that should be included in a balanced eating program. I'm talking here about the natural starches and sugars found in so many foods. These are sources of quick energy, as well as protection against using up the valuable proteins that are needed to maintain the tissues. As this is a new and lifelong approach to eating, your maintenance diet most definitely will have to include all the essentials; however, the carbohydrate as well as the fat intake should be controlled. Carbohydrates are especially needed for tissue repair; without them the body would be using up the protein it should be storing.

Healthful, natural carbohydrates abound in all fruits and most vegetables. The carbohydrates that you should eliminate are such calorie-filled substances as rice, sugar, flour, the products made from sugar-filled jams and jellies, soft drinks, and devitalized foods like potato chips, cold cereals, and any other foods that have been so processed that their original value has been lost. Foods such as these simply clog your system, interfere with proper utilization of good foods, and sit around on your hips. But you can't and shouldn't completely eliminate sugar from your diet. It's best in its natural form, which is glucose. Glucose is needed by the brain for proper functioning: fresh fruit, eaten every day, will keep your energy and your spirits up and is the best way to get your supply of sugar.

Hypoglycemia, or low blood sugar, is a debilitating condition. The blood needs a certain amount of sugar to keep you from being tired and listless. But it doesn't need it from a candy bar or a piece of pastry, which will only give you a temporary lift, as it does not efficiently raise enough blood sugar. Quite the contrary: the temporary lift is followed by a sudden drop, leaving you in worse shape (in both senses) than before.

Natural glucose, on the other hand, stays with the body, giving energy in a normal flow. Remember that, sugar, any sugar, heavily processed as it is, is no good to anybody. Avoid it!

Let me say a few things about *water*. It is mandatory for any kind of diet, be it spot-reducing or long-term. You need water to keep your kidneys active in flushing out toxic wastes from your system. Sometimes overweight comes not so much from overeating as from water buildup—how many people do you know who eat comparatively little but are still overweight? Toxic poisons from undigested food can bloat the body.

Water is necessary for elimination. But there are two things you must bear in mind:

1. Salt retains water in the body tissues, so it's best to cut down on your added salt intake.

2. The more water you drink, the more efficient the elimination process. It's best to drink at least eight glasses of water a day, but, as I have stated before, not during, prior to or directly after a meal—give yourself at least twenty minutes each way.

These two facts may sound contradictory but they are not. The water that you drink on a salt-free or low-salt diet will flush toxins out of your system. However when water is consumed at the same time as food, it interferes with the digestive process by diluting the natural digestive fluids.

A diet based on sound principles will eliminate minor problems that a nonbalanced diet can create, such as constipation. Fresh fruits and vegetables are invaluable for good digestion and elimination, as is a small amount of fat or oil. That's one of the reasons for including these in your diet. Easy-to-digest meals, plus all that water *between* meals, should help you digest, eliminate, and feel fine and healthy.

The maintenance diet will include certain foods which have natural diuretic, or water-eliminating, properties: foods like grapefruit, cabbage, watercress, fennel, apples, radishes and pineapple. And, with a little experimenting, you will find you don't miss added salt at all. Lemon juice can point up the flavor of just about any food from hamburger to melon. If you have never cooked or flavored with herbs, invest in some thyme, rosemary, basil, sage and oregano. Chicken flavored with rosemary rubbed on the skin is unbeatable. Tarragon, basil or thyme sprinkled on salads or in dressings are flavorful accents. A pinch of oregano adds flavor to eggs. And herbs are good for you. Experiment and see how little salt you need.

Because all natural foods have something special to contribute to the body's functioning, it's especially important to keep your diet varied, as I do mine. Enough of all the essential vitamins and minerals naturally found in foods must be supplied each day for maximum well-being. If you become familiar with the important properties of these vitamins and minerals, you will find it much easier to follow the structure of the diet. Here are some of them.

Vitamin A: This vitamin has a beneficial effect on the skin; it keeps it smooth and healthy. It's also essential for the health of your bones and teeth, for good eyesight and firm nails. The best sources are all yellow vegetables, dark green leafy vegetables, liver and eggs.

Vitamin B Complex: While each of the separate components of the B complex is valuable for some specific function, the best way to take vitamin B is as a whole. Each component acts better when the whole vitamin B complex is taken. Vitamin B helps the nervous system to function well, helps the digestive system to burn foods and is useful in forming the red blood cells.

The components of Vitamin B complex are:

B_1 (thiamine): Helps digestion and elimination and promotes healthy nerves. It's found in organ meats (heart, liver and kidneys) eggs, green leafy vegetables.

B_2 (riboflavin): Helps metabolize carbohydrates and proteins, is good for the eyes and helps to calm the nerves. It's also essential for the health of the skin. Liver and kidney are rich sources, as are skim milk, cheese, yogurt, poultry, leafy green vegetables and avocados.

B_6 (pyridoxine): Helps the muscles and nerves to function well, helps in cases of oily skin, and has to do with the formation of blood. Best sources are liver, meats, egg yolks, skim milk and green vegetables.

B_{12} (cyanocobalamin): This is the anti-anemia substance. Best sources are animal foods: organ meats, eggs, fish; also skim milk.

Other components of the Vitamin B complex are:

Niacin: Helps to oxidize carbohydrates. It is found in lean meats, powdered milk, leafy green vegetables and fish.

Choline: Helps to prevent cholesterol buildup. It is found in egg yolks, liver, leafy green vegetables and nuts.

Inositol: Works with choline to protect the liver; helps the body absorb vitamin E. It's found in fruit, also in liver and kidneys.

Biotin: Helps the body to digest and assimilate fats. It is found in liver.

Folic Acid: Important for the formation of red blood cells. It is found in meat and leafy green vegetables.

Pantothenic Acid: Essential for the digestive system, especially for carbohydrate metabolism. It is found in organ meats, broccoli, mushrooms and egg yolk.

Vitamin C: This is a vitamin that the body does *not* store, so you should take some every day. It is said to prevent fatigue. Teeth and gums need vitamin C, as do connective tissues and capillary walls. Vitamin C helps to fight infections. It's found in citrus fruits, tomatoes, leafy green vegetables, potatoes, red or green peppers, berries and melons.

Vitamin D: Known as the "sunshine" vitamin because the body manufactures it when exposed to the sun's rays. Needed for good teeth and bones, and to utilize calcium and phosphorus. Besides the sun, Vitamin D is in fish, fish-liver oil, eggs and skim milk.

Vitamin E: Helps the body to break down fats and to store oxygen. It's found in rich amounts in corn oil and peanut oil, as well as in fresh beef liver, fruits and green leafy vegetables.

Vitamin F: Helps in the distribution of calcium and absorbs the fat-soluble vitamins A, D, E and K. It's in vegetable oils.

Vitamin K: The body manufactures this one, which helps

in clotting of the blood. It's found in all leafy green vegetables.

Vitamin P: Works with Vitamin C and comes from rose hips and all the other sources of C.

Minerals are needed to work with the vitamins and also help to regulate the water balance.

Calcium: Essential for strong bones and teeth; helps to prevent insomnia, irritability and muscle cramps. Found in skim milk, cottage cheese, yellow cheese, yogurt, sesame seed, broccoli and turnip greens.

Phosphorus: It works with calcium, but it needs Vitamin D also. It is found in fish, meat, poultry and cranberries.

Iron: Helps ward off anemia and is vital to the absorption of oxygen by the lungs. Rich iron sources are: liver, eggs, avocados, oysters and leafy green vegetables.

Iodine: Helps keep the thyroid functioning and healthy. The thyroid regulates the metabolism, and thus directly influences body weight. Iodine is in fish, shellfish and kelp.

Magnesium: Very important for elimination. Especially while you are on a diet, proper, regular elimination is a must for good health. Leafy greens, natural unprocessed honey, nuts and clams are rich sources of magnesium.

Potassium: Helps control the body's water balance. Meat, fish, green vegetables, apple juice, fresh and dried fruits and paprika all contain potassium.

Sodium: Maintains body fluids. When you are on a salt-free diet to help cut down on fluids, you will still get what sodium your body needs from such foods as fish, seafood, artichokes and all greens.

Many of my models whom I have put on diets have asked if they couldn't be sure of getting all the essential vitamins and minerals by taking vitamin supplements. I would say that in certain circumstances these can be most helpful. There are times when the food we eat isn't all it should be, due to overcooking, freezing, peeling and other mistreatment of natural foods. But no supplement can give quite the nutritional value of good food, correctly prepared. It's more than worth the effort to have the proper diet. After you have made sure that you have a sound eating plan, there may still be an individual need for extra supplies of some vitamins. Everyone's system is different, and what may be good for your neighbor may not be good for you. I myself take vitamins daily. You may not need to.

What is most important is for you to see to it that your diet provides all the vital nutritional elements, as we have outlined. If you eat all the things you need, if you skip all the junk extras you don't need, you are well on the way to a healthy eating plan.

Protect yourself, your health, your figure and your disposition by getting the most out of the food you eat. You do this by 1: buying only the best quality of foods available; 2: preparing it with care and consideration. Good quality food doesn't need much in the way of flavorings, seasonings or sauces, so right there you are ahead in the calorie count. Buy lean meats, and always broil or roast. Fish is a natural ally to the dieter, low in fat and rich in easily digested protein. Fish, broiled or baked, is marvelous with nothing more than lemon juice or you can use the recipes in my book *A More Beautiful You in 21 Days*. Eggs can be cooked in a Teflon pan, thereby giving you all the protein without any fat added in cooking. Cottage cheese, as you know, is the dieter's best friend, but you can also eat other cheeses, as long as they are not the processed kind. Natural cheese of the low-fat type is a good source of protein and can be used in flavorsome, nourishing dishes.

Learn to love salads. You can keep such salad makings as carrot strips, watercress, raw mushrooms, celery, dandelion greens, fresh young spinach and raw string beans in the refrigerator for between-meal snacks. You can also combine them with such fascinating greens as Romaine, chicory, Bibb lettuce and endive, as well as raw zucchini and cucumbers, to make zesty and filling salads. Combine vegetables for texture and flavor, and you will find you don't need fancy, heavy dressings. Lemon juice will do wonders for your salads. Herbs and a little light oil such as safflower or peanut will help point up the naturally appealing flavors of the greens. When washing salad ingredients, dry them thoroughly, either in a spin dryer or metal basket shaken over the sink, or by gently patting with towels. They will stay crisp and, if you add dressing, will be coated, not soggy, with the added ingredients.

The best sweets are the natural sugars found in fruits. Once you get used to them, diet or no diet, you will find, as many of my models have, that pastries, chocolates, sodas and other so-called goodies are distasteful to you. With your palate re-educated, you will just naturally strike from your shopping list all the forbidden foods, the kind that would ruin your new figure.

Reeducating your palate is the most important part of your program, but there is also the matter of reeducating your other eating habits. We've been brought up on three square meals a day. It's much better to eat small, light meals, and, to avoid hunger pangs, to have light snacks in between. You will find this literally shrinks your stomach, so that it can hold only a small amount of food at a time. You just won't be able to stuff yourself, even if you want to. Put the seal on the good work by chewing all food thoroughly. This, too, will help you to eat less; since digesting begins in the mouth, you will reach the satiation point much more quickly.

Now for the maintenance diet itself, based on all the points that have been outlined. The diet is simplicity itself, and one on which you can ring many changes, all based on the guidelines laid out for you. I have purposely avoided putting rigid restrictions to each meal, since you know enough by now to choose wisely. Here, in outline, is my maintenance diet for keeping the new you:

Breakfast

Fruit or juice. Protein food: cheese, eggs or lean meat. Coffee, black or tea without milk (20 minutes after your meal). Sugar substitute if you haven't learned to drink beverages without sugar.

Mid-morning snack

Fruit or juice, any of the raw vegetables in the salad group: radishes, mushrooms, cucumbers, carrots, for example.

Lunch

Any lean protein food—fish, meat, cheese or poached, boiled or scrambled eggs, if you haven't had them at breakfast. Either raw fruit such as melon or an apple, or sliced raw vegetables, but in very small quantities.

Afternoon snack

Raw vegetables.

Dinner

Soup or vegetable juice—be sure to use the recipes from your Fourteen-day Diet if you enjoyed them as much as I did! Lean protein meats: liver, chicken, lean ham slices, hamburger; or fish. Choose two or three vegetable dishes as side dishes, seasoned with lemon and herbs as you prefer. Salad. Fresh fruit for dessert—better yet, save it for an evening snack time, if you usually get hungry then.

It goes without saying that all portions should be moderate. Fish is the one exception; you can have a little more of that, since it is so naturally low in calories. There are lots of wonderful fish and seafood recipes in *A More Beautiful You in 21 Days*. Still, as part of your reeducation plan, it isn't wise to eat lots of anything, as you stretch your capacity for food. If you should find yourself losing weight after you have gotten down to your desired poundage, increase your daily intake. Once you eliminate your fat palate, you'll be surprised at how much you'll prefer eating a large slice of melon instead of a fat-building slice of pie. You'll also be astonished at your feeling of well-being every day. You not only will feel like doing more, you *will* do more, and enjoy doing it.

5

Keeping the Body Young

If you feel that you've gone as far as you need on the daily fourteen-minute exercise plan for fourteen days—and you're ready to maintain your new figure—then, great! Isn't the human body sensational? All it asks is to be fed properly and to be maintained through minimal exercise.

You don't have to swim a mile a day or jog all over town to maintain what you've got. You don't even have to leave your home to join a gym or health club unless that's what you want. The following exercises done in your own home will keep you in shape forever! They cover every portion of your anatomy and will take a scant twenty minutes a day—the twenty minutes that you might spend telling me you don't have the time. Don't let anyone—child, husband or relative—take this time from you. It's yours, all yours. Use it for your health and beauty's sake.

First you must *loosen the muscles* with these exercises. Do each one for one minute.

1. Stand straight with your feet a little apart, arms hanging loosely at your sides. Keeping your head straight, rotate your

shoulders in a circle. Up, back, pulling your shoulder blades together, down and forward.

2. Stand with your feet slightly apart. Bend forward at the waist with your head hanging down. Make large circles with both your arms at the same time. You will look like a windmill.

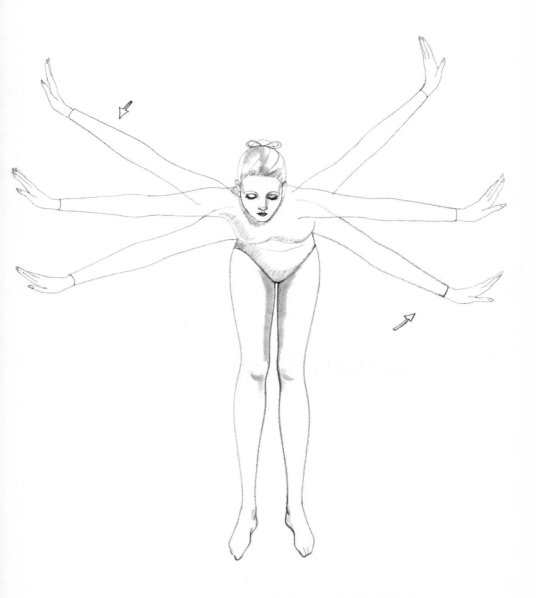

3. Sit on the floor. Bend your knees and pull your heels as close to your bottom as possible. Holding onto your toes, slowly walk your heels forward as far as possible. Your body will bend forward. When you have progressed as far as you can go comfortably, breathe deeply and slowly three times. Walk your heels back, still holding onto your toes. Repeat three times.

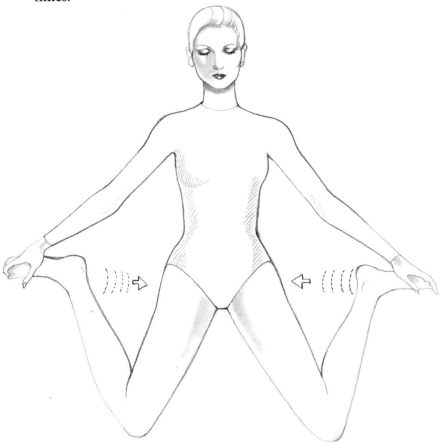

Now continue with the following exercises, which are for very specific parts of your body. Even if you don't think you need them, do them. When you see the results, you will know that you did need them.

4. *For the abdomen:* Lie on the floor. Lift your legs about two inches from the floor. Open and close them scissors-style. Start with two times and work up to twenty.

5. *For the thighs:* Stand like a fencer with your right leg behind you and your left knee bent. Be sure your right foot is pointing straight ahead and that your left foot is pointing a little in. Now bounce up and down ten (working up to thirty) times. Reverse and repeat with right knee bent and left leg behind you.

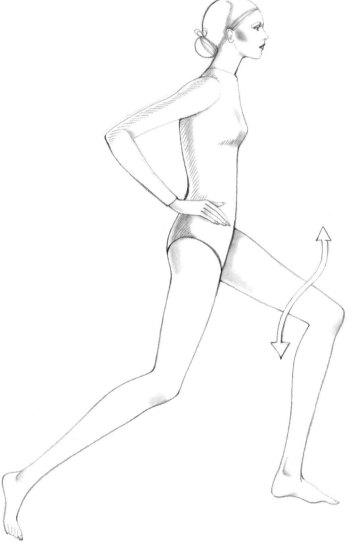

6. *For inner thigh:* Lie on the floor, knees bent, feet flat and about twelve inches forward of buttocks. Tighten inner thigh muscles starting at knees and continuing all the way down. Let the muscles pull your inner thighs as close together as possible. Hold for a count of three and relax. Repeat twenty times.

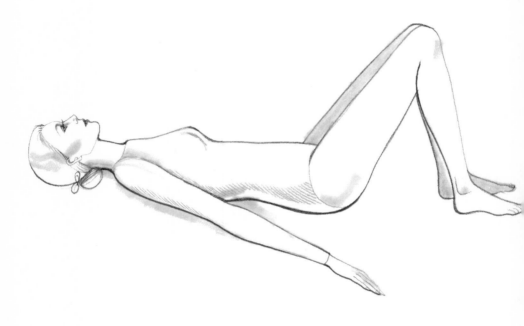

7. *For the diaphragm:* Stand straight, legs together, arms hanging loosely at sides. Contract your diaphragm, breathe deeply, relax and exhale. Repeat ten times; work up to twenty-five times.

8. *For the arms:* Stand erect. Raise arms to shoulder level. Extend arms straight out and back as far as possible. Make little circles to front, then to the rear, keeping outstretched arms at shoulder level. Repeat ten times in each direction.

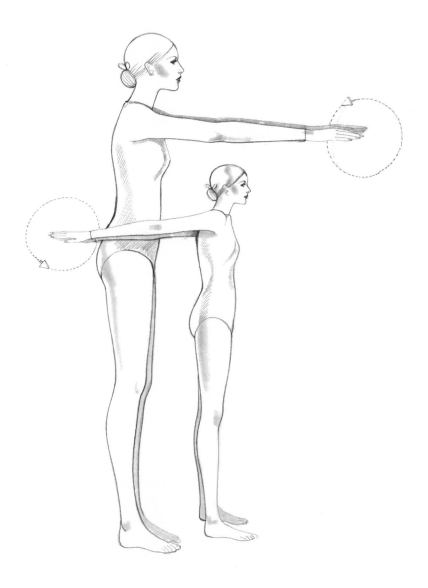

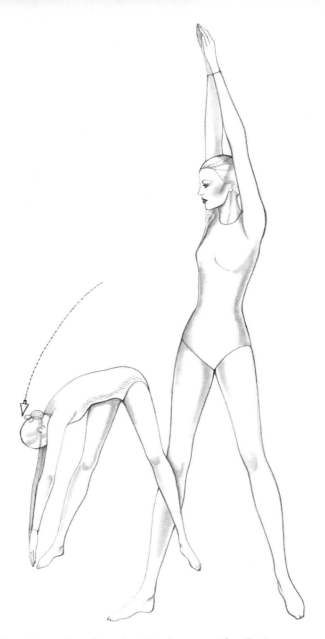

9. *For the waist:* Stand with feet astride. Raise your arms over your head, inhaling as you do. Twist to the right, then bend and try to touch left toe, exhaling as you do. Now repeat, twisting to the left and trying to touch right toe. Repeat five times on each side, working up to twenty on each side. The inhaling and exhaling are very important to this exercise. Be careful not to become dizzy at first, and don't try to actually touch your toes until your body is ready.

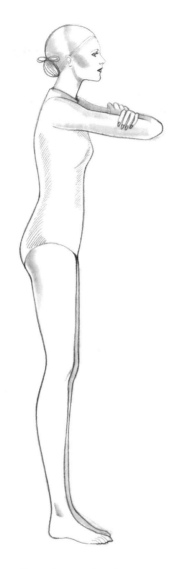

10. *For the bosom:* Stand straight, feet together. Raise arms to shoulder level, bend arms and place left hand on right arm just above the elbow, place the right hand on the arm just above the left elbow. Quickly push hands on arms as if you were pushing up your sleeves. You will feel and see the pectoral muscles at work. Start with ten times and work up to twenty-five.

11. *To get your circulation working:* Start jogging in place, slowly at first, working up to as fast as you can. Start with one minute; work up to ten, if you can. I can never emphasize the value of this running in place. There is just nothing like it for the entire body and mind.

There you have it! These exercises may seem entirely too easy to do the work of maintaining your entire body in top condition. Believe me, they can. Bear this in mind about your body and mind (it's not an original thought): If you don't use it, you lose it. Don't lose your capacity to enjoy life because you didn't exercise. Reject the thoughts of dull brains, memories and hearing as necessary components of the aging process. These are only for the foolish who are literally allowing sloth to promise them a miserable body with an even more dismal future.

Your present and future can be the best that nature has to offer. Are you going to deny yourself the twenty minutes a day it takes to insure them? No, you are not; you've read this far because you really care—care enough to continue today!

6

Makeup Is Forever

I don't think I've ever been interviewed by a reporter who hasn't asked me how faces have changed. The fact is that faces don't change. From Nefertiti to this year's beauty, the defined cheekbones, the wide-set eyes, the long neck, the slender hands, legs and feet, all remain the eternal components of beauty. What does change is the fashion in makeup. There is always a new look for a face, depending on the fashions of the moment, and any woman can look lovely when she uses makeup well to enhance her own individual look.

Women tend to worry too much about their own defects. Tiny flaws become disfiguring to the worrier, when, in truth, the rest of the world will hardly notice them. If it's not a flaw that must be corrected surgically, makeup can achieve miracles for you, providing you play up your assets and minimize the defects. With just a little concentration you can "design" your face.

To design your own face may seem a superhuman task. It isn't, really. It takes time. It takes practice. It also takes several trips to beauty counters to determine exactly what makeup is right for you. Go to the beauty counter with a clean, moisturized face. Try on various bases and wear them to see their effect on your skin. If the color turns, if your skin feels dry from the makeup, if you have any allergic reaction, that makeup is not for you.

This may be time-consuming, but it's the only way. The same principle holds true for blushes, powders and eye makeup: try them, if possible, before purchasing them.

Experience has shown me that as skin gets older, liquid makeup blends more readily and doesn't settle into lines as do powders and cake makeup. The same holds true for color and contour makeup—sticks, gels and liquids blend more readily.

Apply liquid makeup (for that matter, any makeup) over a freshly cleansed and moisturized face. Using your fingertips, blend the makeup upward and outward, making sure you cover enough of the jawline to avoid a masklike appearance. Try to make up with a shade of makeup as close to your own skin as possible. You can add more color with the next step.

I have found a liquid color that contains a moisturizer. I dot it all over my face and blend. The effect is that of a constant suntan, even in the winter. It's a great glow. Then I highlight my cheekbones with a creamy lighter-colored frosted stick.

It is at this point that finishing powder should be dusted over the face. I personally use powder on my nose to keep it from shining and on my lips to keep lipstick from going into the little lines about my lips. An almost-shiny, healthy, glowing effect is what you want to achieve.

If you have problems that you want to conceal, such as a broad nose or puffs under the eyes, remember the rule that light colors bring things out and dark colors make them recede. The special problems that develop with time are puffy eyes, heavy flesh under the brows (see eye makeup, below), sagging chin lines. These can be corrected to a certain extent with makeup. However, for those who feel they are beyond the help of mere makeup, Chapter 9 discusses the matter of plastic surgery.

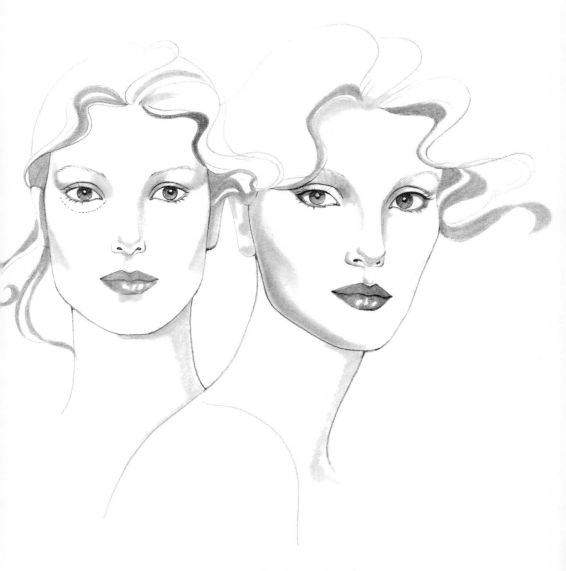

For puffs under the eyes, a shade of liquid makeup base two shades lighter than the all-over base should be patted carefully in that area. Never powder here. Powder will add a dry, creased look that is to be avoided at all costs.

Carefully blend makeup base two shades darker than your own skin color from your earlobe diagonally across the jaw-line to your chin to minimize a chin line that seems to droop.

Eyes are your most individual feature and can, with makeup, be played up as your most important beauty asset.

It all starts with the eyebrows. Remember that they are the frames for your eyes. Even when the fashion dictates, I don't like thin, arched brows. Marlene Dietrich may look great in them or the model on the magazine page may look very "in," but on the rest of us they look artificial and can toughen the whole appearance.

The brow should begin at the inside corner of the eye; the arch should be over the outer edge of the pupil when you look straight ahead in a mirror, and the brow should end at the outer corner of the eye. The beginning and end of the brow should be on the same level.

The color of your eyebrow should be somewhat lighter than your own hair—never darker, unless you have very blond or white hair. Eyebrows can be bleached or dyed the same color as your hair—but be very careful not to get the color in your eyes.

There are so many mascaras on the market today that the choice is bewildering. The lash-thickening mascaras eliminate the need for false lashes. I was at the market the other day and a woman came in wearing heavy false lashes. She really looked old and out of style. The younger customers were convulsed with laughter. Remember that any color mascara except brown and black never did much for your lashes. I'm not even sure the colored mascaras are still on the market. My advice would be to discard any you might have left over so that you won't feel tempted to use it.

The use of eyeliners should be minimal. The line should be drawn close to the lashes on the upper lid with a fine brush or pencil. Eyeliner under the eyes has a tendency to smudge and make the eye look smaller, so stay away from using it there.

The real wizardry of eye makeup is that you can, with the proper use of shadow, change the shape of your eyes—make small eyes large, minimize protruding eyes—the variations are endless. Learning to do the tricks takes time, but the results are so dramatic that it's truly worth the time and effort it takes.

Close-set eyes can appear wide-set by applying a beige shadow in the corner of the eye closest to the nose and then applying a smoky-toned shadow at the outer edge.

Keep mascara away from the little lashes closest to your nose.

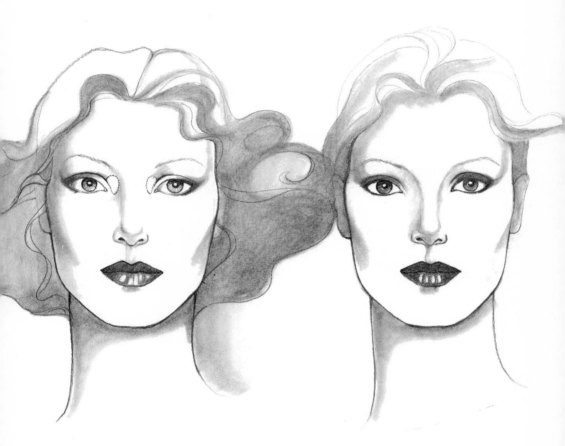

Drooping lids that make you look like a female Robert Mitchum can be made to look less sleepy by widening the eye shadow at the outer corner of your lid and bringing it up just a bit. Use an eyelash curler, too.

Bulging eyes can be made less prominent by using smoky-colored eyeshadow from the inner to the outer corner of the lid in an even arc and using a tiny bit at the outer corner underneath. Then smudge the shadow a bit with a cotton swab or your finger tip.

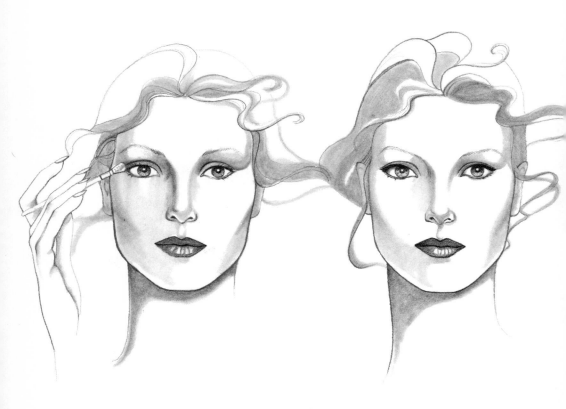

Narrow or small eyes can be enlarged by extending eyeshadow out a tiny bit at the outer corners and filling in between the shadow with beige or white eyeshadow applied with a brush.

Overhanging flesh above the eye can best be corrected by plastic surgery. However, the overhanging brow can appear less so if eyeshadow in a taupe or smoky brown is applied in an arc over the eyelid, with a lighter color applied on the lid itself.

Eyes are enormously sensitive to lack of sleep, dust, pollen and alcohol. There are no oil glands around the eyes so the skin in this area wrinkles more readily than the rest of the face. This all adds up to one thing: Take care of your eyes!

Each morning, as you moisturize, gently pat some extra moisturizer around the eye area. If your eyes are red, use drops. I have found that the constant use of drops is habit-forming for the eyes, so use them only as needed.

In the evening, remove your eye makeup this way: Moisten a cotton square with peanut oil or eye-makeup remover, and, closing your eyelashes over a tissue, gently remove the mascara and eyeshadow, taking care not to get the oil in your eyes.

After cleansing and moisturizing your skin, pat a few drops of peanut oil at the outer corner of your eyes.

Lips are a big fashion point. Old-fashioned colors can date you. Look at what's new in the magazines and use it. There's no such thing as one color lipstick and nail polish for every use. You should have a wardrobe of at least two or three colors and coordinate them with what you're wearing. Your eye makeup can and should be coordinated to go with your lips, nails and clothing, too.

Before you apply your lipstick, powder your lips lightly; then outline your lips with a brush or pencil and fill in the outline with whatever color you have chosen for the outfit you are going to wear. Blot the lipstick with a tissue, powder again and reapply the color. This will make it last longer. Finally, apply a shiny, lustrous lip gleamer. Dry lips never did appeal, but a dewy, moist mouth has been a symbol of beauty since forever.

There really isn't much point to talking about makeup unless you devise a plan that will maintain your skin.

As time goes by, the skin requires ever more constant

vigilance. For some reason, pores can enlarge, and conversely, skin becomes drier and hormone imbalance can cause adult acne.

One thing must be said about skin: that time does precisely nothing to help it.

The nice thing about living now is that there are really incredible choices of beauty aids at the beauty counters. In fact, there are so many that I'm going to try to sort them out a bit for you.

Remember these three basic principles for skin care:

1. Cleanse
2. Refresh
3. Moisturize

These steps form the basis for everybody's skin-care program from here to eternity. The products may change but the formula never. Let's go through a program for daily skin care step by step.

In the morning: Cleanse

1. If you have dry skin, use a lubricating cleanser such as toilet lanolin, Spry or Crisco. You can use your favorite lanolin basic cleanser if you wish; just make sure it contains a lubricant, then tissue off.

2. If you have normal skin, use a soap, if you wish. I use castile soap that comes in large bars; cut it up into small ones and store them in plastic wrap. You can also use a lanolin-base cleanser. If you use soap, remember to rinse until your face is squeaky clean.

3. If you are battling adult acne, wash with a liquid facial wash. There are at least three good ones sold at cosmetic counters. Wash with your fingertips, never with a washcloth, and rinse, rinse, rinse until you are sure it's all off your face. Never use beauty grains—they enlarge the pores.

Refresh

I have never believed in astringents. They are too strong for my taste. Every cosmetic company makes a mild skin toner; or

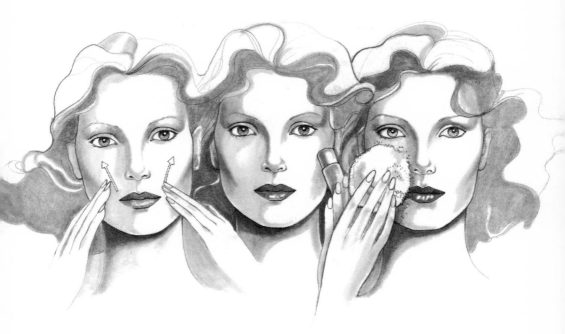

you can pat on witch hazel with a piece of cotton. This closes the pores.

Moisturize

There are a bewildering number of moisturizers to choose from. Oily moisturizers clog the pores. If you can find a hypo-allergenic moisturizer that isn't drying, you are better off. Mine is made by a dermatologist and it's great. However, here we're talking about the principles of skin care, and the important fact to remember is that you must moisturize daily.

In the evening: Daily

Repeat the above procedure with perhaps the addition of patting a tiny bit of peanut oil in the crow's feet around the eyes. I don't believe in throat creams and all those extras that we all hope may help. They won't; all they have ever done for me is take up space in my medicine cabinet.

The only variation here will be if you are affected by acne. The best investment you can make is a facial sauna. You should steam your face nightly until the pores are open. Take a tissue and gently press out the oil in the skin, then wash with your medicated liquid soap. Rinse with cool water until your face is squeaky clean and apply a medicated cream such as a disaster cream on the troubled spots and moisturize the rest. Never use a product that contains camphor; it is far too drying.

Weekly you should plan to give yourself a facial, complete with mask and luxury bath. It may take time, but there's no shortcut to beauty. Each year takes its toll, and the only way to hold back time is to take it and use it for yourself.

Weekly facial
1. Cleanse your skin as you would daily. However, today you should steam your skin with a facial sauna or by letting the hot water run in a basin as you bend over it with a towel over your head until the pores are open. Then take a tissue and gently press out the excess oil that has accumulated.
2. Apply a mask—any mask that pleases you. (I have several that I have acquired through the department-store beauty specials.) Relax in your beauty bath. Finally, remove the mask.
3. Go over your whole face with a cleansing facial brush (unless you have fragile skin) and a little castile soap.
4. Rinse, rinse, rinse—at least thirty times—with cool water.
5. Apply freshener.
6. Apply moisture cream.
7. Apply makeup.

You can tell the difference in the way your makeup looks if you have given yourself a facial. There's a tingly look that nothing else can duplicate.

A word about that luxury bath. Because I work, I shower to save time. Saturday afternoon, however, after I've done my weekly marketing and lunch is over, is my time for a facial and a bath.

The skin on your body deserves the same care as your face. You should go over skin in the tub or shower with a fingernail brush or pumice stone daily, pay special attention to your upper arms, chest, heels and soles; your feet seem to get tougher than other parts of the body. Apply body moisturizing cream all over every time you bathe or shower.

The Saturday afternoon special is something else. I fill the tub with hot water and bubbles and sit back with my mask

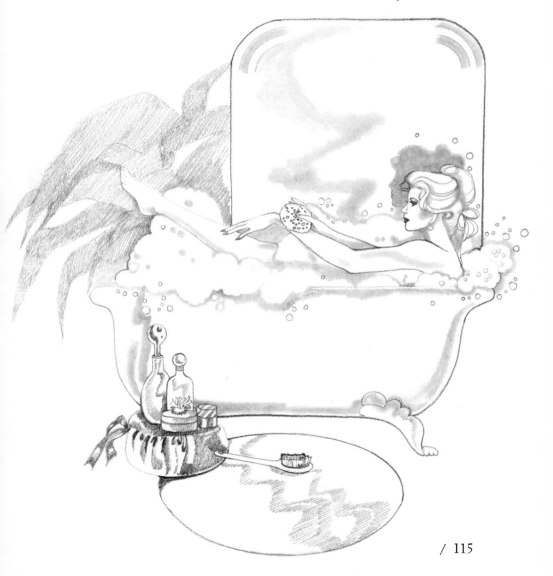

on, a cassette playing my favorite opera, and I relax. I sit until the water begins to cool, then I wash and use the pumice or nailbrush all over my body. The whole bath takes about twenty minutes to a half hour. When I get out of the bath, I remove the mask, finish off the facial and feel that I can face the world again. I am sure that it's the time alone and the quiet, with nothing particularly on my mind, that does the good. We all need that moment of peace, whoever we are.

The program I have outlined is really minimal both in time and effort, for your body, makeup and skin. What you want to achieve is the look of health. Glorious skin, lovely makeup and a body toned to its best all combine to give you that look. It's a combination that can't be beat. You can't have one without the other. So, follow the program I have outlined every day for two weeks. Let the compliments roll in!

7

Hair Care

Fashions change from year to year, but the most dramatic changes always seem to be the hairstyles. As I look back at some of the early pictures of my models, I am struck most by the difference a hairdo can make. Sometimes I feel women don't take as much advantage of their hair as they might. I can't imagine why masses of women would all wear one hairstyle just because it is chic at that moment. Yes, the hair itself may look very pretty, but it won't help to distinguish you from everyone else. It's not doing anything for the woman beneath the hair. That's what I mean when I say that my models can be, and have been, changed drastically and dramatically by what they have done to their hair. You don't have to go to extremes to look different, but you should try to cultivate a look that is uniquely you.

The change does not have to be so obvious that people will say immediately, "Oh, yes, I can see instantly what you did. My, it certainly must have taken a lot of work!" The change can be much more subtle. In fact, it may look like nothing at all. Sunny Harnett, one of the all-time modeling greats, looked as if she did nothing to her hair. She wore a very simple hairdo that looked as if it were the way her hair fell naturally and she had nothing to do with it at all. Of course, with her slim elegance and complete confidence, she could get away with it.

The truth is, Sunny wasn't getting away with anything! It simply happened that her lovely features looked better with simple hairdos than with fussed-over ones. But she paid lots of attention to her hair. It was very fine and required plenty of care. She was careful about its color, its condition and its cleanliness—despite the fact that it looked very casual and above all natural.

I could go on and on about my models and their hairstyles, but right now I'm more interested in you. I not only want to see you become more beautiful than you already are; I'm also going to tell you all the steps you'll need to take. Don't tell me you've worn your hair a certain way for years and you don't think much can be done now. The whole point is that you most definitely can and should transform yourself into a more vital, a more attractive, a more distinguished you. I put great emphasis on that last word, you. Get ready to be more intrinsically, more individually you than you have ever been before.

First, the facts you should know about your hair: Hair is made of various proteins supplied to it by the foods you eat—which is why your diet has so much to do with it. Each strand —all two hundred thousand of them—is nurtured via oil glands attached to the follicle, the pocket in the scalp that holds the roots. The functioning of the glands is what determines the condition of your hair—normal, oily or dry. The daily average loss of hairs is somewhere between fifty and seventy-five, and each hair has a life span of up to two years. Healthy hair goes through this normal cycle of growth, loss and renewal. The steps to better hair care that I'm going to tell you about can vary depending on the oil content of your hair.

Begin by investing in a natural bristle brush, which will spread your hair's natural oils thoroughly. A nylon brush is just not as effective. The best way to brush is by standing with your head bent downward so that you're actually brushing from the back of your head to the front. Aside from distributing the oils evenly, this has two purposes: First, it cuts down on hairs falling from the crown of your head, its most sensitive area; and second, it leaves your hair with a natural tease so that you won't have to worry about putting in added height. Be sure to brush your hair especially well at night to remove any dirt or tangles before you go to sleep.

Because circulation is important in hair growth—hair needs all the oxygen it can get—I recommend a daily fingertip massage to get that scalp alive. Put your hands on each side of your head, with your fingers spread wide. Gently rotate the scalp. For further increase in circulation, do this simple exercise at mid-point in your day: Let your head drop forward, slowly turn to the left side, to the back, to the right side, and repeat. This relaxes the nerves and any constriction in the scalp.

The next step involves finding the correct shampoo for you and using it properly. Shampooing is a good protective measure against the daily damage caused by the environment, especially in large urban areas. For normal hair, choose any product you like—a castile, herbal or protein shampoo is good. Because of its degreasing properties, a lemon shampoo is excellent for oily hair: be careful not to buy a shampoo with merely the lemon fragrance; look for a product containing real lemon. Read the ingredients: if they aren't listed clearly, look for a different brand of shampoo. For dry hair, choose a product with a lanolin base. When shampooing, rub with the fingertips—not the nails—carefully and firmly into the scalp to remove dead cells: never scratch your scalp. Rinse and apply again. When rinsing, start with warm water and graduate to cold, particularly if you have oily hair, as this will tighten the pores. When you're sure you've rinsed out all the suds, do it again. Without a mirror, it's hard to see spots you may have missed, and a dry coat of suds on the hair will leave it with a dull film. A balsam rinse is beneficial to dry hair; a solution of lemon juice and warm water to oily hair.

Now let's talk about conditioning. Normal hair should get that special treatment once a month or once every two months. However, hair that has been exposed to the sun and has become dry and brittle will need more frequent applications. Look for a deep-down conditioner that remains on the hair for at least twenty minutes; above all, avoid excessive use of hot rollers, which only dry the hair out more. For really damaged hair, I recommend hot oil treatments that you can either buy or receive at a salon. The easiest way is to warm some olive oil in a saucepan and apply it into the scalp after sectioning your hair. Wrap the entire head in a hot towel and sit for fifteen minutes, changing the towel as it cools off. Then shampoo thoroughly. This treatment gives the hair luxurious body and a great sheen.

Here are some other tips for protecting the hair. If you have long locks, it is best to condition them more often than the rest of the head to avoid split ends. Also remember to wash hair immediately after bathing either in a chlorinated pool or in salt water during those sunny months that do the most damage to both hair and skin. If you have a special problem, discuss it with your hairdresser—if you don't have a hairdresser, write to the beauty editor of any fashion magazine.

More and more salons are making a specialty of having at least one hair-and-scalp-conditioning expert in the house. He will concentrate on getting your hair into sleek, shining condition before even thinking of a style. Your hairdresser will soon get to know what you need in the way of hair care. He will take an interest in the condition of your hair, as well as its styling, if he is at all good.

Trichology, the analysis of the hair shaft and its follicle, is no longer found in only the exclusive beauty centers. Trained trichologists will soon be in many shops, and your hair needs will be scientifically determined. Treatments will then be based on the information gathered from the individual's scalp condition. Most experts have their own preferred treatments, concentrating on *releasing* the scalp to work its own natural processes of feeding and revitalizing the hair.

One treatment that hair experts seem to use as a common denominator is a relaxing massage of the scalp, shoulder and neck area. I have tried them and they are miraculous. Not only did my hair show more life afterward, but I felt relaxed all over. Even my voice sounded softer and less tense! That goes to show you how interlocked all our physical processes are.

Trichologists take their profession increasingly seriously as the field becomes more and more competitive. They have been developing individual formulas to speed the recovery and reconditioning of damaged hair. Interestingly enough, they devise their formulas out of natural materials, such as fruit and vegetable juices and herbs. Chemicals have ruined enough hair; what it needs is honest-to-goodness protein. You'll be experiencing the newest of techniques. Whichever expert you choose, you can be confident that you will emerge with a better head of hair, more amenable to any new style you might want to try.

If your problem is dandruff, it's best in most cases to get rid of it yourself. Steam your scalp with hot towels. Use a medicated shampoo, allowing it to remain on the scalp for several minutes before a super-thorough rinsing. It takes a little more time and effort than the usual shampoo, but it really works.

Another problem has to do with thinning hair. As I said before, it is normal for as many as seventy-five hairs a day to fall out. But you may find that my tips on brushing and maintaining aren't curbing excessive hair loss. Let me explain why, so you'll know what you may, or may not, expect.

Dermatologists are agreed that hair normally gets a bit thinner with age. Unless your follicles, those pockets that hold the roots, are damaged, a hair will start growing back as soon as one falls out. There are, however, many things that can affect the follicles, dermatologists have discovered. For one thing, it's known that the predominantly male hormone called androgen, found also in women, has much to do with hair loss. There are many things that affect the production of androgen, though nothing has been pinpointed for sure.

Likely causes are emotional stress, hormone imbalance, vitamin or mineral deficiencies. All seem equally possible.

Great emotional stress has the effect of increasing the production of androgen, and it is this disproportional output that sometimes causes loss of hair at menopause. At the other extreme, taking the birth control pill can have this same effect because it also causes a hormone imbalance.

The thyroid gland, too, may have a lot to do with it. An over- or underactive thyroid condition can easily affect hair production. Any one of a number of nutrition-related deficiencies may be the cause, so a visit to your doctor may prove helpful. Only he will be able to diagnose such a problem.

There is hope for thinning hair, so don't despair. Dr. Norman Orentreich, who has pioneered in so many fields relating to hair loss, is working with drugs that may counteract androgen. He feels that there is definite hope for prevention and cure of baldness in the near future. For the present, Dr. Orentreich has developed a procedure of transferring small plugs of hair from one's own scalp from an area where it is plentiful to another part of the scalp where the hair doesn't flourish.

Fortunately the emphasis on the importance of hair has encouraged all kinds of research and treatments. They are expensive; but if you are desperate, consult your county medical society before choosing a doctor.

It's time to start thinking about enhancing the hair. Most of my models have chosen coloring to do this. My personal feeling is that hair coloring is on a par with makeup: most of us could use a little help. The proper coloring on your face makes your features come alive; and the same thing happens with your hair. Sometimes just a shade of difference will bring out your looks to an astonishing degree.

Don't think I am saying that all women must color their hair. There is the question of temperament to be considered. I knew a girl of eighteen who had gone heavily gray and who decided to keep her hair that way. She felt it gave her a certain distinction. Her youthful, piquant face under those gray curls was arresting. Of course, she kept her hair in meticulous condition. It is my own belief, however, that though it did make her look startling, it made her look a lot older too.

An older woman whose gray hair is carefully tended and becomingly coiffured is truly beautiful. If she is comfortable with her hair, that is all that matters. I find my appearance improved with regular hair coloring, since those gray streaks do nothing for my morale or my looks. You may want to join the growing sorority of color-at-home women, or you may want to entrust yourself to the hands of an expert at a salon. In either case, follow-up care will require a certain amount of discipline on your part.

Once your hair is dyed or bleached or rinsed or whatever, you are *committed* to keep the color ever fresh. Your schedule has to include a definite time for touch-ups. The natural color of the roots should never be allowed to show. Hair that has been colored needs to be pampered. Artificial color can be ruined by too much sun; swimming without protection for your hair in either a pool or salt water will only damage it further. Keep your hair covered in bright sun—there's no other way of shielding it.

Before you choose a color, you must consider the natural color of your hair. It will affect the final result of the coloring, especially if you use a rinse rather than a dye. If you have very dark hair and want to become a light blonde, you must first have your hair stripped of its natural color before it is dyed blond. Your hair will have to be tended very carefully from then on because the stripping will inevitably give it a certain fragility, and unless you are very handy, it's really difficult to do yourself.

If you want to add red highlights to your tresses, that's easily done with rinses. Don't, however, fool around with straight henna. If you prefer henna, go to a professional hairdresser. Henna packs have to be very carefully timed and mixed. This is especially true if you have gray in your hair because if improperly applied it will make those strands turn a bright orange. Even a professional has to keep a careful chart of the formula he has worked out. A touch of red is devastatingly lovely; a touch too much will just be devastating. I can't emphasize too much going to a professional for this. God's truth, I'm not a henna fan, so to me it's *all* devastating.

You can lighten or darken the tone of your hair easily enough if you stay within your natural shade range. A mousy brownette can become a warm auburn or a vivid brown or a dark blonde. I have known natural blondes who have slightly darkened their hair as they got older; they felt they had a bleached-out look that was more appropriate to younger girls.

Almost any shade of dye or rinse should be fine, except for black. Black dye has a tendency to look like just that: black dye. To be perfectly frank, it isn't too flattering to women over twenty-five.

Along with your natural hair color, you must also consider your other coloring before you select a new hair shade. It is most important to find a color that will play up your eyes. If you have green eyes, for instance, you will look smashing with the right auburn tone. Blue eyes don't necessarily have to go with blond hair; a warm brown shows them up too. Dark, dark eyes can be complemented with a dark brown shade of hair. Gray eyes are made even prettier with a light russet head.

Also, consider your skin tone. If you have the sort of skin that tans easily, don't try to be a redhead. If you have dark or sallow skin, don't try it either. Keep your hair in a darker shade. You can have blond highlights—in fact, you should see to it that your dyed hair isn't all one color: natural hair color isn't one color, either. Fair skin looks lovely with blond or reddish hair. A soft medium brown is very becoming to almost everyone. It may not be as dramatic as other shades, but you will have more leeway in choosing makeup and clothes that won't clash.

It sounds as though I've given you many warnings, but it's because I want to give you the quick route to a more beautiful you. You can experiment, but I want you to avoid time-consuming procedures. To help you get the best results, you should understand the differences in the products available.

Hair coloring products come in two basic forms: one is for temporary coloring, the other for permanent. The effects of each are also very different. Temporary color comes from color rinses and color shampoos. Both are really meant for bringing out highlights, not for changing the natural color of your hair. They cannot make dark hair light, and the rinse will effectively darken only blond hair. Misusing a rinse in the attempt to get a new color will result in a streaky mix of the rinse color and your own. Rinses are good for the woman who simply wants to enhance her own color, and, since they contain no peroxide, will give your hair only a minimum of dyeing. It is also comforting to know that if you don't like the result, it can be washed right out.

With permanent dyes the process gets more complicated. I prefer the aniline dyes over the metallic and vegetable types— that tricky henna is one of the latter—because aniline dyes will not interfere with any other processing you might want to do later. It also offers four different methods to choose from, depending on how much change you want: highlighting shampoo tints, shampoo-in tints, one-step dyeing and two-step dyeing. Highlighting shampoo tints will give you virtually the same effects as the temporary rinses will, but because the "permanent" dyes contain some peroxide, the highlighting lasts up to six shampoos. Like the temporary kind, they also will not cover gray. The shampoo-in tints contain even more peroxide and thus enable you to go several tones lighter or darker than your own shade. Again, after six shampoos or six weeks, the color will need renewing. Either of these products are easy to use, and with a little practice you should be able to do it yourself with ease. For colors that require one- and two-step dyeing, I strongly suggest that you let your hairdresser do the work. As you will see, the processes are quite tricky.

One-step coloring lightens and colors at the same time, but though your choice of shades is greater than with the tints, you still won't be able to go from very dark to light blond shades. However, you will be able to cover gray completely.

Two-step coloring is the most difficult and damaging to the hair. If this is the only way for you to achieve the color you want, then be prepared to give your hair intensive care, or else it will become brittle. Two-step coloring does two things: first, it removes the natural pigment from your hair; second, it replaces it with the color you desire. It takes well over three hours to complete the entire process. As you can imagine, three hours' worth of various chemicals are going to take their toll on your hair. On top of that, maintenance, which involves coloring the roots every six weeks, will leave the hair that is close to the scalp the most brittle of all. In this kind of coloring, the steps to take after the dye has been administered are as important, if not more so, than the dye job itself. You and your hairdresser should work out a schedule of hair care that you can follow through at home. This must include protein conditioners and shampoos. Those hot oil treatments I mentioned before are excellent too. You can see why it's best to have a professional behind you.

If you've really got your mind set on blond hair, but are a little apprehensive about the effect it's going to have, why not consider frosting your hair? The process is similar to that of two-step coloring, but because you are only coloring a few selected strands, you won't have problems with roots or excessive brittleness. A little frosting on brown hair will brighten your whole head very beautifully.

Now that you've got the color you want, it's time to consider a style. Just because you've been wearing the same one for a while now doesn't mean you shouldn't or can't change. One of the most frequent complaints I hear about hair is that it's either too curly or too straight. Well, if you feel that one of these is your hair problem, let me tell you that it doesn't have to be a problem for long. Straightening and permanent waving are being done in the home as well as in the salon these days. And if you should want to do it yourself, it takes only a little patience and experience to do it well.

Straightening and waving use the same principles: Break down the molecules that hold the hair in its natural shape and reorganize them so that your hair will be straight or waved. Incidentally, both processes use the same chemical lotion. The difference is that in the first it's combed through, and in the second it is used with rollers. Touch-ups for either depend on the length of the hair and on the growth rate. If your hair is short and frequently cut, the process will have to be repeated more quickly than it would if your hair were long. Again, you should be extra considerate to your hair by using the right shampoos and by conditioning often.

When it comes to the actual question of styling, remember that a jewel deserves a perfect setting. You should look as lovely as you are. And just as a jeweler studies every facet of a gem before finding the right setting that will enhance its beauty the most, so should you find the hairstyle that is most becoming to you.

Stand in front of a full-length mirror. Check out your dimensions. Tiny and small-boned? Tall with small bones? Medium all around? Are you broad-shouldered or big-hipped? Believe it or not, all this does make a difference, because what we're considering here are the overall dimensions to be complemented by your hairstyle. A small-headed woman with a small hairdo on top of a broad body is out of proportion. A tiny woman who tries to foster the illusion of height by one of those towering hairdos only calls more attention to her small stature.

If you are tiny, make the most of it. If you are tall, play it up. If you are broad-shouldered, let your hair come out a little from the sides to help soften your proportions. Of course, the way you dress also has a lot to do with the way you will style your hair.

Consider the way you live. Many of my models, who are busy women, wear their hair very simply. True, they must usually have their tresses styled for the camera, but these are not the coiffures of their choice. I, too, dress my hair very simply. I am always in the middle of ten different projects; nevertheless, I have to look well at all times. I imagine that you would also prefer a hairstyle that is attractive but not time-consuming to achieve. When you are going to a party or a special evening is planned, you may want a high-fashion coiffure. Just make sure it becomes you. Consider the shape and contour of your face to bring the whole picture into focus.

If you have the perfect oval face—lucky you—play up to it! Don't hide your jawline with droopy hair. You can wear your hair brushed back from your face, or with a middle or side part. If you have pretty ears, show them; enhance them with a simple pair of gold earrings to complete the picture.

A long, narrow face can be made to look fuller via width. You may want to wear straight short bangs or little tendrils around the crown. Brush hair as much to the sides as you can. A side part, with the fuller side brushed a little up and outward, is a good device.

If your face is too round, keep your hair up off the face, adding some height. If you have long hair, pull it back and finish off with a high French knot or chignon. If your hair is short, try a part that starts far off to one side of your head but forms a diagonal line as it goes from the center of your head to the back. That way you can cut the width by letting a single sleek wave cover most of the crown.

If your face is on the squarish side, keep your hair off the jawline. A small amount of height at the crown and fullness to round out the ends will make your face look slimmer.

A heart-shaped face can be balanced by keeping the top of the hair sleek and creating fullness below the ears.

Your hairdresser will have some helpful ideas of his own. You should try to get your hair professionally done at least once a month. Your hairdresser can discuss styles with you for the other weeks at the same time. I think that more and more salons are happy to work with women on this basis, rather than pushing some new pet style of their own. It helps them too, by building a following of clients. He can discuss any of the processes available to you and help you choose what is best for your individual type of hair.

While we're still on the question of styling, I want to put in a word about wigs. Many women find them indispensable. I think that they should be used and treated with care, as if they were your own hair. There is more than just the obvious difference between falls and wigs; what they do should be taken into account.

A full wig presses down on the scalp and cuts off its natural breathing process. My suggestion is to save wigs for the times you want to be a totally different you, or when you are just plain in a hurry and simply don't have the time to do your own hair properly. Speaking of which, you should never be seen with a sloppy or dirty head of hair; it's unattractive and unhealthy. Hiding it in a scarf constantly is not an answer; save your pretty scarves for those special looks. One warning though: Don't tie them too tightly or, like wigs, they will interfere with scalp circulation and leave your hair dull and lifeless.

My preference, if you need to add fullness to your own hair, is to use a hairpiece such as a fall. This is attached with hair or with bobby pins crisscrossed against each other. A hairpiece gives your scalp plenty of breathing space and gives you a great deal of freedom. You can have a lot of fun with a hairpiece, changing the style of your hair at will. It goes without saying that you should find the perfect match for your own hair in both color and texture.

Now that I've told you how to get your own personal, utterly new style, don't be afraid to change if the mood strikes you. Your hairstyle should be as versatile as you are. After all, the whole point here is not to get into the rut of one hairstyle or one shade of lipstick. The essence of life is change, experiment and growth. You'll never make a mistake that can't be corrected. So feel free to be you!

8

Trips for Beauty

I know that we can't stay young forever; yet heads of state such as Churchill and Adenauer—and Tito as a current example—continued their direction of nations until the end of their eighties, their minds clear, their bodies functional, like men thirty or fifty years their junior.

As sophisticated as I may be about beauty and beauty spas, I didn't know that these distinguished people, and myriad others all went (Tito still alive and well) to health spas. These spas are to be found all over the earth, but the most outstanding seem to be in Europe.

It's fine to contemplate being young and full of the zest for living, with our mental forces at their peak, for the rest of our days. But it takes time and money to go to beauty and health spas. Oddly enough, the beauty spas cost more than those dedicated to giving us a continuing life force. If you have the money, it's worth it. If you would have spent the money on a vacation in some resort anyway, you might consider a visit to a spa as a vacation. Your money will be better spent at La Prairie, for instance, than on a boring, fattening cruise. Once all our children are educated and we, hopefully, will have some extra cash, we both hope to try these spas.

As I say, some spas are beautifiers only; some are more medical in their approach. For me, where there is health, there is beauty and I don't need to go anywhere to learn about makeup and other beauty aids, so I would opt for the health spa. You may want a beauty spa more than an out-and-out health spa; the choice is up to you.

In order to make that choice, you should know about the places that are being run especially to bring about the optimum state of health for you—a state in which you will just naturally glow from within—and about the people who run them. In addition, there are many that will teach you all the refinements of outer adornment. There you will learn about makeup and carriage and style—all designed for you and you alone. Because that's what a true beauty is—she is her own best, unique, individual self.

There are so many spas, it's hard to know where to begin. I'll start with the basic type—the health spa. Health spas have been around longer than civilized man. Primitive peoples, often more versed than civilized ones in natural healing and beautifying processes, have known for centuries that certain parts of the earth had some natural property that would bring back health and grace.

There is a place in Mexico, a beach in San Blas, Nayarit, where the Indians practice what we would call "spa cures." They come down from the mountains and dig holes quite close to the water, burying themselves in the sand, leaving only the face uncovered. Then someone pours sea water by the bucketful over the sand-buried Indian. Fifteen minutes to half an hour is all it takes. They say the sand packs have marvelous curative powers for nervous conditions and blood disorders. A scientific explanation might be that the mineral properties of the sea, absorbed via the mud bath, effect the healing. The point is, it works.

There are spas oriented toward the curative properties of mineral baths in most European countries. We have some in the United States, too—for example in Saratoga, New York, and in Florida. There used to be many more. I think it's terribly sad that such a simple and effective method of treating ailments to which we are all subject is disappearing. I personally would like to see American spas reactivated for the benefit of us all.

There is a spa in Germany called Bad Pyrmont (*bad* in German is spa) which is near Hanover. The spa is state-owned and operated, though there are many individual clinics. According to the brochure published by the state government and approved by the State Medical Association, diseases of the heart and circulation can be treated there. Anemia and rheumatism are also treated, as well as women's hormone disorders, eczema, allergies, exhaustion and diseases of old age.

The explanation is simple. Mineral waters, such as those found at the spa, have curative powers. There must be something to it; people have been coming to the spa for two thousand years!

Spas don't depend on only the waters. Doctors who have made studies of what can be done in such surroundings have set up clinics with medical staffs to further the good effects of the waters. As an example, there is the sanatorium of Dr. Buchinger situated at Bad Pyrmont.

Among the offerings at the Buchinger Sanatorium are massage, mud baths, herb-tea scrub baths, saunas. He also conducts supervised fasts, using the therapeutic effects of the mineral-rich waters, along with vegetable juices and teas. The sanatorium claims excellent results in such disparate conditions as high blood pressure, skin disorders and rheumatic disorders.

There are spas and clinics that go even further in their use of natural substances for healing. Where they don't have the natural curative substances of mineral springs, many spas and clinics turn to the earth, in the form of good food—fruits, vegetables, honey, goat's milk. Landlocked Switzerland has the clinic of Dr. Max Bircher-Benner. He maintained that raw foods contained a "life force," a quality of nutritive energy or sun energy that was lost in foods subjected to chemical tampering or heating.

More and more scientists are doing research into the health-giving properties of foods, and we who live in this scientific age should be grateful to them and heed what they say about the foods we eat.

The doctor believed in *living* foods, foods that are fresh and vital, formed out of nature's own forces—sun, soil, air and water—filled with what he called *matière vivante*. It was this living material on which he relied for his cures, many of which were termed miraculous. He pioneered in the use of fresh juices, fresh salads, fresh green leaves, the "sun-cooked" foods that contain the most life-giving energy.

If you go to the Bircher-Benner Sanatorium in Zurich, Switzerland, you may well find your life will never be quite the same. First, the very atmosphere is calming, soothing, revivifying. The sanatorium is on a beautiful hillside overlooking Zurich, and those Swiss panoramas are a treat in themselves. I, for one, can't look at a scenic view without experiencing an instant, indescribable peace. The soothing effect on my soul finds an answering response in my body. The surge of peace, of new energy, gives me a respite from whatever problems, mental or physical, have been nagging at me. It's nature's restorative, and it is free for the asking. Try to find some serene, green place, steep yourself in the oasis of peace and life-giving sunshine, and you will be renewed. That's the first step.

The sanatorium compounds all the goodness in the atmosphere with the use of nature's pure abundance. The health and beauty diet there is a simple one. The "living" foods are served up in simple, appetizing form: fresh vegetables, milk, mounds of green salads. Here, too, is the origin of the famous muesli. In case you can't get to the sanatorium, here is the original recipe.

Muesli: Mix a level tablespoon of oatmeal (you can use another cereal if you like) in two tablespoons of water and soak overnight. When you are ready to eat it, add the juice of half a lemon and a tablespoon of condensed milk. Stir. Shred a large unpeeled apple into the mixture, stir in a tablespoon of honey and another of wheat germ.

That's it. It's delicious, nourishing, energy-giving and re-vitalizing, they say. I can't bear it.

You can't possibly know what a miracle-working regimen this simple diet can be until you've tried it. Naturally, at the clinic everything is prepared from the freshest foods obtainable. This is half their value. The foods still contain the enzymes which have so pronounced an effect on the body. By virtue of these fresh and freshly prepared foods, the digestive system is given a chance to cleanse itself of accumulated impurities and toxins. That means not only helping to rid the body of diseases; the healthful effects of these foods on the normal body are seen as well. A more shapely figure, better hair and nails, and glowing skin color come naturally with good health.

I have said that Dr. Bircher-Benner was a great modern pioneer, and he was indeed. But the concept of using good fresh foods is as old as medicine. It was Hippocrates who said, "Let your food be your best medicine."

More than two thousand years ago it was another Greek physician, Diocles Carystos, who said, "Eat raw fresh foods first of all, eat cooked foods as the second course, and let fruit be the end of your meal."

Was there a real reason for this? Good food in any form is good food. Some time back there was a scientist, Dr. Rudolf Virchow, who found out *why* you should eat raw foods first. To put it briefly, he observed that eating cooked foods at the beginning of a meal called up an increase of white corpuscles in the blood. This is the "immune reaction" that the body makes to disease germs and bacteria. It is the body's self-protection device. For some reason, the body wants to protect itself against cooked foods when they are eaten as a first course. When fresh raw foods are eaten first, there is no "immune reaction." Cooked foods can be eaten as a second course with no untoward effects.

We are fortunate to be living in an age when new ideas can be so quickly spread. People whose business is primarily beauty rather than health have been wise enough to see the value of sound health practices. There are many "beauty spas" today that use a combination of health and beauty disciplines to teach a woman how to cherish herself.

People respond to you in the way you think of yourself. You should think of yourself as someone worth caring for. One of the great values of beauty spas is their emphasis on just that. The investment makes for happy returns, in looks and health —and in inspiring those around you to greater love.

There are so many of these wonderful places that will take you in hand, give you diets, massage, show you how to exercise and make up. And *how to relax*. So many of us need to learn how to unwind, how to take stock of ourselves as human beings. We aren't "wasting time" when we relax, as some people seem to think. We are recharging our energies in the best way possible, by getting in tune with our natural forces.

Here is the sort of reconstructing, revivifying program you will find at these beauty spas.

Elizabeth Arden's Maine Chance, Phoenix, Arizona. Personal pampering is the core of this 105-acre establishment, though at first pampering might not seem quite the right word. The day starts with breakfast in bed, which softens the fact that what you get for breakfast is decaffeinated coffee with a sugar substitute, grapefruit and melba toast.

The velvet glove treatment goes on like that all day. The surroundings are not merely elegantly luxurious—they are soothing as well. You are surrounded by original art (Chagall, Georgia O'Keeffe), polished marble floors, exquisite china and linen, elegantly appointed salons, and, outdoors, by perfectly tended grounds and fantastic views of Camelback Mountain.

But you do have an active daily schedule, all devoted to the end result of making you beautiful. It goes like this:

A.M.
9:00   exercises
9:30   steam cabinet, sauna, warm bath, or whirlpool
10:00 massage
11:00 exercise, perhaps in the swimming pool
11:30 face treatment
P.M.
12:30 hair and nails
1:00   luncheon
2:30   makeup class
3:30   exercise

All the while, of course, you are learning what to do for yourself so when you go home you will be able to follow the program that has been specially tailored for you. Besides the exercises, you learn such beauty secrets as how to massage your scalp, how to care for your skin, new tricks with makeup and how to care for your hands and feet.

One of the most important lessons at Maine Chance is getting acquainted with diet menus that don't taste like diet menus! On 900 calories a day, here is a sample of what you can eat:

BREAKFAST
    fresh grapefruit
    decaffeinated coffee, black, sugar substitute
    unbuttered melba toast
MID-MORNING
    cup of beef broth
LUNCH
    platter of cottage cheese surrounded by fresh fruit
    salad dressing made of plain yogurt and honey
AFTERNOON
    glass of fresh grapefruit juice
PRE-DINNER
    fresh vegetables—carrot sticks, green pepper slices, raw
    cauliflower, etc., served with salt substitute
    tomato juice cocktail

DINNER

baked chicken
spinach ball
cauliflower and cream sauce
low-calorie strawberry-flavored gelatin
decaffeinated black coffee

Prices run from $800 to $1,100 for the week, which runs from Sunday to Sunday. Write to: Reservation Office, Maine Chance, Phoenix, Arizona 85108 (phone 602–947–6365).

The Greenhouse, in Arlington, Texas, is run by Neiman-Marcus and Charles of the Ritz. As one would expect from this combination, the latest in luxury is the key here, but underneath the Southern comfort is a lot of knowledgeable discipline. The exercises are devised by Toni Beck, a professional choreographer and dance teacher, who has also written a book of exercises following many of the precepts she had laid down at the Greenhouse. The diets are devised by Helen Corbett, who was formerly with Cornell Medical Center, is now consultant to Neiman-Marcus Food Services, and has written *Cook for Looks*. As in Maine Chance, you can either lose or gain weight, depending on your needs.

The daily schedule goes like this:

A.M.
8:00   Breakfast in Bed
8:30   Wake-up Exercise
9:00   Swing and Sway the Greenhouse Way
10:00   The Beautiful Facial
11:00   Water Exercise
Noon: Modern Makeup Mastery
P.M.
1:00   Luncheon
2:00   Hair Styling, Hand and Foot Care
2:30   Spot Reducing
3:00   Sauna and Needle Shower
3:30   Massage
4:30   Rest and Dress

<pre>
6:30   "Cocktails"
7:00   Dinner
</pre>

For a little mental stimulation and entertainment after dinner, The Greenhouse invites special guests, an assortment that might include an astrologer, a yogi, a wine expert, a fashion expert. The Greenhouse will also, if you like, take you into Dallas to shop at Neiman-Marcus.

Meals that appear to be sumptuous but are actually slimming are served around the famous pool in the high, luxurious solarium, or in the formal candlelit dining room. They add up to no more than 850 calories a day, if you're slimming down, but are imaginative and delicious. Here's a sample:

BREAKFAST
    grapefruit
    homemade soybean and wheat germ bread
    coffee or tea
10:00 A.M.
    potassium broth (celery, carrots, parsnips, etc.)
LUNCH
    small cheese soufflé made with extra egg whites
    salad
3:30 P.M.
    sugarless fruit ice
5:00 P.M.
    yogurt or gazpacho
DINNER
    roast veal with lemon

Makeup techniques, face care, hair styling, manicures and pedicures are under the direction of the Charles of the Ritz salons. You learn how to keep up the good work once you get home. You can also take home a copy of your diet.

The week is Sunday to Sunday, and the price is $825, plus 15 percent service fee in lieu of all gratuities. Write to: The Greenhouse of Neiman-Marcus, P.O. Box 1144, Arlington,

Texas 76010 (phone: 214–261–8221). I've never been there, but it is said to be great!

The Greenhouse also offers special services. The Silver Spoon caters to young women in their college years. Couples, obviously for husbands and wives, has a special program of exercise and grooming for men. The Mother-Daughter program is—well—for mother and daughter.

The Golden Door, Escondido, California (Highway 395, Escondido, Calif.), one of the most glamorous of the beauty spas, is run along substantially the same lines as these others. They too will send information by mail.

If you'd like to combine foreign travel with your stay at a beauty spa, here are some outside the United States:

Beauty Farm, Knebworth, Hertfordshire, England. This place has moderate prices and is reputed to be very efficient.

Clinique Diététique, Champigny, France. This is a converted country house that specializes in physiotherapy as well as diet and exercise.

As you can see, the idea of combining the forces of health and beauty is growing. I am looking forward to the day— which may not be so far distant—when a stay at a beauty spa will be as much taken for granted as a day at the beach.

An even further step in the use of nature's forces to revitalize us involves a scientist who carried to a daring conclusion the discovery of other scientists. Paul Virchow did much research on cells. Did you know that each one of us is composed of forty trillion cells? Each cell is a living, separate organism. We are supposed to be constantly renewing these cells in our bodies. Virchow called the cell the "Life-Bearer." Just consider this—all these trillions of components of our bodies, living and transforming themselves.

Virchow and others claimed that sickness of the cells was the forerunner of sickness of the whole body. With that as a premise, Dr. Paul Niehans came to the conclusion that fresh, healthy cells from young animals could be used to replace the ailing cells of human beings. He used nature's own nourishment to heal, to youthify and to beautify.

La Prairie, his clinic in Switzerland, has for years treated via cell therapy the rich, the famous, and others who had ailments, or those who simply wanted to hold on to their youth a while longer. Sexual rejuvenation, of course, was a popular pursuit. But Dr. Neihans' work involved more than that. I have heard of a famous beauty expert who got rid of her migraines via Dr. Niehans' cellular therapy.

Niehans felt that he could work wonders for weak and tired people who could now "refresh themselves at the living sap of cells."

I confess it gave me a bit of queasiness to realize that what was involved was cells from unborn lambs. Logically, I suppose it's no more to be deplored than some of the protein foods we eat; heaven knows baby lamb chops are a great delicacy. Thousands of people have had heartening results with Dr. Niehans' therapy. Somerset Maugham, for one, regained his failing powers after visiting La Prairie and started to write superb stories once again.

Dr. Niehans has passed on, but his theories and his work are more alive than ever. You can still go to La Prairie, a charming retreat on Lake Geneva, for fresh-cell injections. Dr. Walter Michel (who was himself cured of paralysis, caused by a car accident, by means of cell injections) now runs the clinic. Treatment takes a week, and the price is around $1,600. A candidate for the treatments must first take tests to determine whether or not cell therapy can be of help. If it can, anywhere from five to ten injections are given; the process itself takes little time.

Many countries in Europe, particularly Switzerland, West Germany and Italy, have doctors who will prescribe cell therapy. Britain and the United States still don't recognize Dr. Niehans' work. If you don't want to go to Europe, you can go to Nassau, in the Bahamas. There Dr. Ivan Popov runs a health spa called Renaissance, something on Dr. Niehans' lines.

Dr. Popov doesn't treat organic illnesses. He is, according to his brochure, more interested in "helping the mature individual counteract the pressures . . . of contemporary life . . . problems of weight, anxiety, and premature aging. . . ." I would imagine that in Nassau it's a little harder to come by as many sheep as roam the Swiss mountainsides! At any rate, Dr. Popov uses freeze-dried cells instead of fresh.

I don't know whether or not Dr. Ana Aslan is one of those whose work takes up a part of Dr. Niehans' discoveries. One spectacular case which Dr. Niehans treated was that of Pope Pius XII, who had been suffering from a diaphragmatic hernia. Other doctors advised an operation; Dr. Niehans advised Novocain. His reasoning was that this would relax the diaphragm. Then, Dr. Niehans said, the Pope was to have lots of mashed potatoes, the bulk of which would liberate the temporarily strangled parts of the stomach.

The Pope followed Dr. Niehans' advice. He lived, without benefit of the operation.

I tell this story only because it involves the use of Novocain as part of a medical treatment. Dr. Ana Aslan makes no secret of the fact that her treatments, which may be in either pill or injection form, employ procaine, which is better known as Novocain.

But her pills and injections contain much more. Again, she makes no secret of her formula, which is called Gerovital H3. The buffered procaine, she says, acts directly on the brain and central nervous system; they can, she claims, make protozoan cells grow. The formula also contains benzoic acid, as well as potassium, which, she says, accelerates the action of the procaine on the heart and brain. Potassium is also one of the most needed elements in nutrition.

Dr. Aslan's formula, for which people gladly travel to Bucharest, is said to be used by one out of ten Rumanians. I wouldn't be at all surprised, since it is apparently a true wonder-worker. Gerovital H3 is said to make for lasting changes in the body. According to D. Aslan, her formula "can strengthen all the senses, make skin blotches vanish, help balance blood pressure, restore hair, even give hair back its natural color."

Gerovital H3 apparently does many things for many people, all of them good. Sex problems are only one area in which it has been useful. Lillian Gish, that remarkable actress, has said that it gives her more energy. Certainly Dr. Aslan herself is a prime example of the energy that Gerovital H3 is said to generate.

She has been taking her own medicine for the last twenty-one years. At seventy-five, she looks a couple of decades younger, works sixteen hours a day, and evidences a quick wit and, most important, concern for every one of her patients.

If you want to try Dr. Aslan's treatments, you have the choice of going to her clinic at Otopeni, Rumania, which is moderately expensive, or at the Institute for Geriatrics, which is downright inexpensive. If you stay at Otopeni, you will have the advantages of other treatments, with hydrotherapy, physiotherapy and electrotherapy offered. The standard fare for health-seekers, as far as diet is concerned: simple foods, mostly fresh fruits and vegetables from the clinic's own gardens. All rooms at Otopeni, incidentally, open onto some section of the large landscaped gardens. You can also stay at her Snagov clinic, a summer place on the Black Sea, which also offers beautiful natural surroundings.

Once you have been to Dr. Aslan, there is no problem about continuing the treatments. You take home a two-year supply of Gerovital H3, together with a form for both Rumanian and U.S. customs certifying that you have been a patient of Dr. Aslan's and need the drug for continuing treatments. Though Gerovital H3 is available throughout most of Europe, it's not officially available in the U.S. Besides the shots and pills, Dr. Aslan also has a cream which is used for skin conditions.

Sharing this particular segment of my researches with you has been one of the most satisfactory experiences I have had in writing this book. It's good to know we can take steps to stay young and vigorous and delighted in life long after the number of years that so many people, unfortunately, take for granted will be dreary ones. We should not only live long lives, but healthy, happy, enjoyable lives. I bless the scientists who have been doing research to this end, and I am sure that they are but the vanguard of a whole movement. I think that in the years to come all these aids to beauty and health and longevity will be taken for granted by everybody. That is what I want to see.

Even if you are young and vigorous, remember that these spas are not only for the aging; they prolong youth in the young and should be considered by all.

There really is a fountain of youth. It's up to you to find it, and when you do, believe me, you'll be glad you did.

9

The Easy Way to Beauty

Everyone asks me, am I going to get a face-lift? The answer is
yes. When the time comes that I feel I don't want to see a
crepy neck or a sagging chin or drooping eyelids, I'm going to
a friendly plastic surgeon and have the condition corrected. I
honestly believe that if the need arises and the money is available, all of us, men and women alike, should contemplate
whatever help is available to us surgically.

I further believe that too-large or too-small noses, breasts
and jaws that damage a person's ego should be corrected, just
as one would correct protruding teeth. Why not? Why should
anyone go through life with a correctable defect that in any
way lessens his self-esteem?

I'm not saying that you must rush out instantly and have
yourself made into a replica of a model. I know that slight imperfections can and should be used to enhance the individual.
For instance, when Lauren Hutton came to the agency, I
advised her to have her teeth and nose fixed. She made it a
point not to get around to it. She cherishes her "banana
nose," as she referred to it in a recent *Vogue* magazine inter-
view, and she uses mortician's wax to hide that distinctive gap

in her mouth. For the camera she is perfect; for her own special lifestyle she is perfect, too. She plays up these minor imperfections to keep her own identity.

On the other hand, one of my newest models, a breathtakingly beautiful girl, is convinced that she needs plastic surgery. She thinks her absolutely beautiful face needs a new nose, among other features. She can hardly be talked out of instantaneous plastic surgery.

These two examples express completely opposite inner feelings toward one's outward beauty. How we feel about ourselves is really the key point here and the single most important factor in determining if surgery is desirable. You should think twice—more than twice—about any advice given to you concerning changing your nose, your breasts, your derrière. Advice from outside may be well meant, but it is not necessarily good. Nobody can know how you really feel; nobody can have a completely unbiased opinion as to what decision would be best for you. Even your best friends can only look at you from their own point of view. They won't have to live with the consequences of your choice—you will. One phrase in the English language that should be ignored is "If I were you . . ."

It is only when you look at yourself critically in the mirror and see a flaw that can and should be corrected that you should start considering ways and means. If the flaw in your face is one that can't be corrected by makeup, or your figure fault can't be exercised and dieted away, then it is time to call on our modern fairy godmother, the cosmetic surgeon.

There is no reason for a nose alteration or the removal of a birthmark to be more acceptable than other cosmetic surgical procedures. The face-lift, for instance, is no longer only for exceptional women, like actresses and rich dowagers. So if you should decide that's what you want, don't feel that you are doing something to cause raised eyebrows—you are not.

The classic face-lift, called a rhytidectomy, is usually given under a local anesthetic. It's an operation in which art is as much called for as is surgical skill. What happens during a rhytidectomy is this: the surgeon makes an incision in the scalp, a little above where the widow's peak is located, if you have one. The incision continues down toward the neck hairline. The skin is then separated from the subcutaneous tissue, precautions being taken by the surgeon not to injure the nerves, the muscles or the large blood vessels. This tissue is gathered up toward the ear and sutured to the fascia, the tissue that protects the facial muscles. Because this fascia is loose and inelastic, the sutures have a tightening effect on it; this causes the face to be "lifted." The excess skin is then removed, more sutures are applied to close the incision, and a firm dressing wraps it up tightly. Generally the sutures are removed after ten days.

In the hands of a skilled cosmetic surgeon, a rhytidectomy truly remakes the face. That is to say, it restores the face you had when you were younger and your muscles firmer. The basic contours of your face will be the same as they were originally; a face-lift will make them resurface. Some women say that it takes a while to get used to a face-lift, since the facial muscles, which had been drooping gradually over a period of years, suddenly tighten up. The adjustment to the unfamiliar firmness does come eventually. A word of warning here: As with any surgery, side effects are to be expected, so take them into consideration. After the operation, sedation is necessary for the first few days to promote smooth healing. Every precaution will be taken to keep your face as still as possible—this includes a diet of liquids, sipped through a straw. You will be mildly uncomfortable for the first couple of weeks, and it will take about a month for all the swelling to go down. Still, they say there's a price for everything. And, monetarily speaking, the face-lift alone can run anywhere upward of a thousand dollars, depending on the physician.

If you aren't ready for, or feel you don't need, a total lift, there are many lesser procedures open to you. Facial surgery of one kind or another can correct almost anything you feel needs fixing, any feature that is less than desirable. Beautiful eyes can make a plain face simply stunning, and there are many operations that can help them look their best. Blepharoplasty is the operation done on the eyelid—whether the top (droopy) one or the bottom (pouchy) one.

You can see what you would look like with the upper lid lifted by cutting a strip of surgical tape and very gently and carefully applying it after pulling up the skin at the temples. This will lift the eye and make it seem youthful and open. You might even wear the strips one evening with a hairstyle that conceals them. I personally think that too much reliance on the strips will eventually cause the skin around the temples to stretch, aggravating the problem.

During the operation on the upper lid, excess skin is removed and the resultant tightening of the area lifts the eyeline. Blepharoplasty on the lower lid will remove those little pouches along the lower lashline. The problem lies in the amount of skin and fat to be removed from either lid; too little or too much can be disastrous. The results of this operation, as well as the others, depends on the skill of the surgeon. The eye operation, whether it is on the lower or upper lid, is performed under a local anesthetic; it takes only a couple of hours and there is only one noticeable side effect: Black-and-blue marks that last for a few weeks. Prices run, on the average, from $400 to $750.

If your major concern is with those wrinkles or frown lines between the eyes that may have become very deep, you might consider silicone injections or a process known as electrocoagulation. The latter is much like electrolysis, the process that removes unwanted hair: tiny electric needles smooth out the wrinkles. You don't have to enter the hospital for this procedure; it can be done in the doctor's office, and the amount of time and the number of visits depend on the amount of work that needs to be done.

Many women may not agree with Sophia Loren, who once said not to change your nose, but, rather, learn to enhance your eyes. For them the answer is rhinoplasty. This operation builds a different nose and must be done with due regard for the proportions the face will assume when the nose is reshaped. A strong-featured face, for instance, really shouldn't have a small nose. If the nose is strong or not absolutely straight, yet in good proportion to the face, a conscientious plastic surgeon will recommend that it be left alone. You don't want to destroy the balance of your face.

It's possible that most noses should indeed be left alone. With all the techniques of makeup at your fingertips, it's easy to create flattering shadows and planes that will remodel the nose. Again we come to the subjective factor. I know a number of women with a perfectly good nose who think it is too long or too short or too something. It's your choice.

I am being so emphatic about this matter because so much of your face's symmetry depends on the nose. On the other hand, because of this factor, it might really be an advantage to have the rhinoplasty done.

Because it is so important to keep the relation of the nose to the face in correct proportion, this operation is done under a local anesthetic; a general anesthetic usually brings on more bleeding, and the face has to be kept as natural-looking as possible for the surgeon to best judge positioning. The operation itself is relatively simple. The surgeon works inside the nose to correct the shape, so there is no outward scarring. If the shape of the nostrils has to be changed, then there will be two tiny scars—hardly noticeable.

Noses can be narrowed, shortened, tilted or straightened. Sometimes surgery to correct a deviated septum is performed at the same time as reshaping the nose.

Plan to stay in the hospital for five days, during which time you will be wearing a nose splint. It will take several months, possibly up to a year, for the healing to be complete. But rhinoplasty is so common these days that people don't even bother to hide out while waiting for the initial swelling to go down.

Less common than the nose "bob" is the nose buildup. This is a little more challenging, but it can be, and has been, done successfully. The surgeon dissects a pocket in the bridge of the nose. Then he inserts an implant, sized exactly to fit the pocket. Again, this is done inside the nose, without any visible scarring. The implant can be from your own rib cartilage, though some surgeons prefer silicone. The healing time for an implanted nose is slightly longer than it is for the shortened one.

Prices for rhinoplasty range from five hundred to a thousand dollars and possibly higher, depending, as always, on the amount of work done.

One of the most dreaded signs of age seems to be the advent of the double chin. Oddly enough, this condition occurs frequently in young girls. But then it is not so noticeable and not so frightening, somehow, as it becomes when we get past forty. A submandibular lipectomy is what may be needed here. This is the operation otherwise known as a chin correction, and it can take one of several forms. If it is a simple question of fat directly under the chin, an incision is made in one of the creases under the chin. The fat is then trimmed away and the incision closed.

If the chin fat extends to the sides of the jaw, it becomes more of a remodeling job, since that fat has to be removed as well in order to keep the face in proportion. Sometimes the chin itself must be corrected. I have heard that Marilyn Monroe was a pretty girl with one little problem—a slightly receding chin. She had a silicone implant and became a beautiful girl.

The chin-reshaping operation is often done along with the one for fat removal. It is one of the most dramatic of all the cosmetic-surgery arts. It requires a close study of the relationship between the skull and the jaws, the length of the bones and the disposition of the teeth. All the art of the surgeon is brought into play here! Only after much careful study and evaluation can he begin to sculpt your new face. And, since the surgeon works inside the mouth, there are no major visible scars. He will probably discuss the subject of dental work during the consultation preceding the operation. Since the positioning of the teeth have much to do with the shape of the jaws, some work may be required in that area. In my opinion, it's never too soon or too late to correct your teeth. I have seen people whose whole faces have changed for the better when they had teeth extracted, replaced or realigned. It can make all the difference in a face. Even ears that protrude can easily, effectively and painlessly be set back.

As I have said, a face reshaping is a work of art. It can make you more beautiful than you thought possible—but it must be looked at objectively. We are often too critical of our looks to make the correct decision about changing them. We ought to look at ourselves with a little more love. But if we still honestly feel that we need some reconstructive help, it's good to know it's available.

The very newest facial surgery techniques, however, are not in face shaping itself, but in the area of complexion enhancement. Very often it is not wrinkles that mar one's appearance —these, as I have told you, can be removed by electrocoagulation—but rather damage done to the skin by acne or other skin conditions. The most standard process for alleviating such conditions is dermabrasion. This means exactly what it says: an abrading of the skin. No, don't be startled. An extremely fine steel-wire brush is rotated at incredibly high speeds to gently scrape away the surface layers of the skin. The scars, blemishes and fine wrinkles on the very top layers of the skin are whisked away by the brush. With healing, the new skin emerges, fresh and blemish-free. Depending on the number of treatments, dermabrasion can run from five hundred to a thousand dollars.

Since this particular technique works only on surface blemishes, the surgeon or dermatologist will first make a careful study of the skin to see just how deep the blemishes go. What dermabrasion can do, it does miraculously. Obviously, if the trouble is more than skin deep, just taking off the top layer of skin won't help.

If you have six weeks or a couple of months to spare, you might want to try chemosurgery. The advantage of this is that the new skin revealed by the surgeon's hands will keep its smoothness for several years. You must follow doctor's orders, however. Most doctors advise that you stay out of the sun and shun liquor and smoking for some time after the treatment.

Chemosurgery uses trichloroacetic acid to burn away the top layer of skin. It is, literally, surgery with chemicals. A hospital stay of two days is usually required. I have seen the results of chemosurgery, and they are remarkable. In the case I saw, the upper lip, so prone to age-giveaway wrinkles, was smooth and young, as was the rest of the face. If you have the patience and an excellent surgeon, chemotherapy can be valuable.

I am most amazed at what is being done by cryosurgery. Cryosurgical operations usually do not require a hospital stay. Only if you have a major skin problem will you be required to stay in a hospital. The results are quickly achieved. What happens is that liquid nitrogen, at sub-zero temperature, is applied by a high-pressure spray to the blemishes, freezing them. The freezing destroys tissue. The top layer of the skin crusts and is eased off. Surgeons have found cryosurgery of value in removing warts and birthmarks, as well as other lesions. I should also tell you that cryosurgery has been valuable in removing skin cancers and cervical cancers. This I call truly miraculous!

There are some beauty institutions that will do facial peeling, but only if it is very light. Usually they have trained and careful operators. For a very light removal of the top skin layer, this peel can be valuable.

A really simple way to alleviate wrinkles is to use silicone for smoothing out facial contours. Some surgeons like silicone; some don't. Still, because I feel you have a right to know all about the new discoveries in instant beauty, I'm going to tell you about it, with pros and cons.

Dr. Norman Orentreich, clinical associate professor of dermatology at New York Medical Center, has been experimenting with silicone for years. He is enthusiastic about its possibilities. What is needed, according to Dr. Orentreich, to utilize liquid silicone for greatest effectiveness and safety, is patience—lots of patience. The surgeon must release the silicone a mere droplet at a time, placing the sharp needle exactly where planned, with a total knowledge of the skin's capacity to absorb in different areas. Dr. Orentreich feels that a competent surgeon can remove wrinkles and fill out skinny spaces esthetically. I have had it done and am very happy with it. However, Dr. Thomas Rees, who is associate professor of clinical surgery at the Institute of Plastic and Reconstructive Surgery of New York University Medical Center, is not so enthusiastic about silicone for the face. He has a point: You can fill in the expression lines on a person's face, but the lines will inevitably be back unless the pattern of the facial expression can be changed. Dr. Rees does use silicone, but for only severe facial disfigurements.

Lately I have been hearing more and more about women who have had a new body sculptured for them by the surgeon's scalpel. At first it didn't seem possible, but then again, why not? If you can reshape the face via surgery, why not the body? The art is not yet as widespread as that of the face-lift, but certainly, as more and more surgeons practice and refine the procedures, it will be more widespread.

I believe that diet and exercise and correct posture should be the first resort of every woman who cares about her body. But I am also perfectly aware of the hard fact that sometimes nothing but surgery will cure certain defects—for instance, heavy, sagging breasts.

In one private clinic in Rio de Janeiro, a Brazilian surgeon daily performs miracles—which to him are routine—on tired, sagging bodies. Dr. Ivo Pitanguy, professor of plastic surgery at the Pontificia Universidade Católica and director of his own clinic, is enthusiastic about perfecting the human body. Dr. Pitanguy will help a woman to achieve her greatest potential with anything from blepharoplasty (eye lift) to tucking in sagging abdomens or smoothing down outsize thighs. And he isn't just touting his own surgical specialty, either. He is known to exhort his patients to diet and to exercise. Especially before an operation, he feels, a patient should lose as much excess weight as possible.

There was a time when plastic surgeons hesitated to operate

on sagging buttocks because previous methods left unsightly scars. Dr. Pitanguy has perfected a technique to correct this. A single flap of adipose tissue is pulled upward and backward to the inner thigh. This neatly lifts the buttocks and smoothes out the thigh at the same time. The advantage in Dr. Pitanguy's procedure is that the scars are not exposed, even when you wear a swimsuit. In fact, these scars tend to grow pale with time, and often, when helped along by massage and exercise, they disappear.

Certainly a firm, slim line of hips and buttocks is worth attaining; to me, surgeons like Dr. Pitanguy are a blessing to the world. I should mention that he really does live up to his ideal of making all women look beautiful. Naturally, most of his clients are very well-to-do, but I have heard that he will also help those who cannot afford the entire fee.

Though he treats most parts of the body, he doesn't like to remove excess fat from the arms. There is no way, he says, that this can be done without leaving visible scars. But who knows? Maybe some day. . . .

In the meantime, he also reshapes flaccid abdomens into nice firm ones with low, narrow, barely visible scars. To those of us who like smooth firm lines and don't seem able to reshape ourselves with diet and exercise, this procedure might be the answer.

Mammaplasty has been left for the last in this discussion; but it is an extremely important and sensitive subject. I don't think there is a woman alive who doesn't have some special feeling about her bosom. She may think the shape too large, too small, that her breasts aren't high enough. Small-breasted women sometimes feel deprived, feel that they aren't "sexy" enough. All I can say to that is, none of my models are terribly full-breasted, and no one is going to tell me that they aren't attractive sexually, as well as in every other way! Men may talk all they like—and some of them do—about the attractions of large breasts, but I have never known any of them to spurn a woman who has small breasts. There's some sort of mystique about the big bosom. But that's all it is—a mystique. One of the nice things about being small-breasted is that you are more apt to keep your firm lines as you grow older.

Don't misunderstand me. *La belle poitrine*, no matter what its size, is a prime attraction in a woman. If she is generously endowed, she is indeed fortunate. Small or large, there is nothing to match the sexual and esthetic appeal of a proudly held bosom.

But then, of course, not all breasts are perfectly formed. Some breasts *are* disproportionately small or disproportionately large. There are mismatched bosoms. There are pendulous breasts, the kind that make bra straps cut into the shoulders.

There are also, fortunately, surgical techniques to correct these and other anomalies. Not only Dr. Pitanguy but other comparatively young surgeons are developing new techniques for reshaping breasts. The United States, Europe and South America all have brilliant, dedicated surgeons who can make breasts smaller, fuller, more symmetrical.

Years ago, silicone was very popular for making smaller breasts fuller. When it was found that liquid silicone had a tendency to wander, leaking out of the breast into other parts of the body, surgeons started looking for other methods. Today silicone is still used, but in different form. Dr. Thomas D. Cronin, of Baylor University in Houston, Texas, devised a much safer method. A gelatinous silicone is sealed in silicone rubber envelopes shaped like breasts. These are inserted into a pocket, prepared by the surgeon, where the mammary gland contacts the chest muscles. The body tissues send out little bits of fibre that enclose the implant.

There is another way of implanting silicone. Small, empty silicone envelopes are inserted into pockets and then a minuscule tube feeds sterilized liquid into the empty silicone pockets.

Surgeons who use the balloon implants claim this method is better, as it leaves smaller scars as well as allowing more control over the size of the implants.

The augmentation technique, in either form, is supposed

to be relatively simple. It would be up to you and your surgeon to choose which method would be best in your particular case. I think a careful, concerned surgeon would be happy to explain to you in detail exactly how he goes about the operation, exactly what cosmetic results you have a right to expect, and whether or not there will be any conspicuous scars. Then it's up to you to make the decision to go ahead or not.

Mammaplasty, in general, is still a relatively young art. That's why the doctors who have developed the techniques are themselves still relatively young and still practicing surgery. Many have evolved brilliant methods that can be followed by other surgeons. Mammaplasty, developed in the twentieth century, will probably be one of the leading beauty aids of the coming decades. You don't have to be terribly young and wearing monokinis at the beach to want full, beautiful breasts. *Any* woman deserves them, and possibly can have them.

Of course, there can be too much of a good thing, and many women have breasts that are simply too big for comfort. Dr. Pitanguy has addressed himself to this very problem. It's admittedly more complicated to reduce the size of breasts than it is to enlarge them, but it is being done. If you are genuinely uncomfortable with your breasts, check into all possible procedures. A hospital near you that has a first-rate plastic surgery unit can describe the methods practiced by their surgeons. Bear in mind that very heavy breasts can be a medical as well as cosmetic problem. Incidentally, I know a nineteen-year-old beauty who could not model because her breasts were too large. She finally decided that she would have her breasts reduced. Today she does many magazine covers and is ecstatic at the result of her surgery.

First-rate work is readily available in the United States. If you need it, avail yourself of it. Prices for breast augmentation start at $500 and go to upward of $750; breast reduction starts at $750 and goes to above $1,500.

I need hardly caution you that once you decide on any kind of remodeling operation, for any part of your face or body, you should shop very carefully for the surgeon. Your family doctor may be able to help you, or possibly a friend who has had successful cosmetic reconstruction. The leading hospital in your city or community might also provide information.

Once you do find a good surgeon, you still have a little more exploring to do. You are certainly entitled to preliminary visits with him. You are also entitled to let him know what you want and expect from him. He should be frank with you about what he can and can't do. A good surgeon will not try to rush you into any snap decision. After all, he is building his reputation on his results. Only when you are satisfied that your questions have been answered fully should you entrust yourself to his skill.

I hope I have given you some idea of how many alternatives are available for the quick road to beauty. I don't think that a healthy, attractive woman should leap at the chance of making radical changes in her anatomy just because she wants to be "perfect" or have some fun. I know some women who can't find enough places on their bodies to change, and I feel sorry for them. On the other hand, if there is a real problem that any of these procedures can solve for you, then go ahead— that's what they are for. Everyone wants and needs to be healthy and attractive. We must make every possible effort to achieve that goal.

10

Change Your Mental Attitude

There are many women alone today. It may be by choice, or due to some other circumstance. The way the woman alone lives her life can be either a rich, fulfilling experience or a miserable withdrawal from all the pleasure of living.

I've heard from women all over the world the age-old cry that "life is passing me by." I know lots of married women who look at single women with more than a bit of envy, and single women who have never married who look at married women with a touch of yearning. I know happy widows and sad. I read every day about mothers who have deserted their families. All of this implies one thing: Women are searching for something—and whether or not they find it is entirely dependent on the way they make themselves fit into society. Even if a woman is single, she still has to make relationships with others in order to find fulfillment. This is the only way to know true happiness.

You can't divorce yourself from life. You can't say, because you have lost your marriage partner by death or divorce, that you have nothing left. If you've never been married, you still have a life to live. Your relationships just take a different form, that's all. If it's nothing more than being pleasant to your neighbors, you have made your presence felt. And, in return, something in you has been marked.

As long as you're breathing, your life isn't over. Of course, things do not remain the same. The essence of life is constant change. If you feel you've never lived, consider that you'll never be any younger than you are now. So start now.

There's a very interesting paradox in the life-without-a-man syndrome. Many such women, whether or not they're conscious of it, feel they are somehow worthless, living alone. They either resign themselves or they go to enormous lengths to make themselves attractive and pleasing to some man—any man. On the other hand, the women who are self-sufficient, with a pleasant sense of their self-worth, usually find that men —nice men—can be found not only in the vicinity, but often on the doorstep. These women find themselves with the pleasant choice of whether to accept one of these men, or not to accept any at all and go on living happily by themselves.

Nobody can make the choice for you. Do you want to go on by yourself? Do you want to share your life, intimately and closely, with one man? Whichever way you choose, there is one thing that is absolutely certain: You are entitled to the very best that is to be found in the world. I'd like to show you how to get that best for yourself.

You are, you must understand, entitled to have the best, simply by virtue of being here, alive, on this planet. Just being created has given you that option. When you exercise your option, you get what you want. Start out by wanting to be a first-class *you*.

Too many women "don't like to bother about themselves." It's not worth the trouble. They get into slipshod ways; they let the dishes pile up, they eat dinner out of a container; they don't give themselves pedicures or manicures or set their hair. They simply don't care. But think of the end result of this pattern of being. I don't say "living"—it's just existing. If *you* don't care about yourself—why should anyone else?

Give up that image of yourself as being alone, forsaken, unworthy. Alone or with someone else, you are most definitely a worthwhile person. You have something to offer. You are uniquely you; no one else in the world has the qualities that you have. Just as you feel that you need someone, don't you think there is someone, somewhere in the world, who needs *you?*

Don't hold yourself back from the world. Perhaps you feel there are many reasons for you to be tied down—you have obligations, commitments, that keep you from being able to get out and make new friends, attract new men, find a new life for yourself.

Let's take that and turn it around. The divorcee, for example, has several real problems. She may have to work, possibly for the first time in her life. If this is your situation, make an opportunity of it! You have a chance to do something you've never done before: To get out into new surroundings and develop new aspects of your personality—possibly to try your hand at something you've always wanted to do but had given up thinking about.

Do you want to teach? Suppose your education doesn't qualify you to give academic courses. These days *everything* is being taught. If you're good at handicrafts, teach that. You will find young, eager pupils flocking to your door. Art? Photography? Whatever you like to do, can you turn it from a hobby to a teaching skill?

You say you can't do anything? Nonsense! One young divorcee with a small daughter wasn't ready to spend her life baby-sitting. She particularly wanted to dance, to do ballroom dancing. She didn't have the money to spend on lessons. So she went to a dance studio, applied for a job as an instructor, and was trained by them. She danced, she enjoyed herself, and she was paid for it. (It should also be mentioned that one of her pupils eventually became her second husband, and a beloved stepfather to her little girl.)

Schooling, groups, courses, are one of the pleasantest and most effective ways of meeting new people—by which I mean men. Cinderella sat behind the kitchen stove and sighed to go to the ball, but I'm afraid that we have to get about if we want to meet the Prince. There are plenty of men out there, and the most exciting are the ones who are *doing* things. They're engaged in business, in research, in the arts, in politics. Many of them are as lonely as you are. Why let the poor things pine away from lack of companionship—yours?

If you take a class in anything, from copywriting to etching, you will still be meeting other adults. And some of them will be men. They are taking the courses to improve their jobs, their opportunities, their minds. *Those* are the men you want to meet. True, many of them will be married. Some of them won't be. And they're as anxious to meet a nice woman as you are to meet a nice man.

If you don't find a man in the class, there are still two new paths to travel, resulting from your education. You may find yourself a job in a new capacity; and there again are the kinds of men you want to meet. Or you may make friends with any of the interesting women you are bound to find in class. Friendship is invaluable. Don't be one of those women who "don't get along with other women" or "don't trust other women." Good friends among your own sex can help broaden your personality, give you support in times of anguish (and we all have those!) and sometimes give you down-to-earth advice, sharing their experiences, to help you through a tangle you couldn't get through alone.

Besides, they know men you don't know. They have brothers, uncles, acquaintances, who to them are merely old and good friends. To you they can be something different.

There was a young widow who was too involved in her demanding job and demanding twelve-year-old daughter to get around much. She made a close friend of a woman who was a divorcee, but on quite friendly terms with her former husband. Yes, that's right: The young widow met the former husband, and believe it or not, they all lived happily ever after. The widow was a little uncertain as to what her friend's attitude would be, but that lady just shrugged and said, "I don't want him myself. Why shouldn't you have him, if that's what you want?" It really turned into a happy marriage and a lasting friendship.

A large part of your meeting new men will depend on your attitude. You can't go around looking as if you're eager to make the acquaintance of any man who comes down the pike. Any man you attract that way will either be out for what he can get from you or be sorry for you. Widows and divorcees are, most unfairly, supposed to be fair game for any man. The widows and divorcees I have known have been quite the opposite. Divorcees, especially, carry around with them a terrible sense of failure. I have talked to many, and they all assure me that it takes about a year to get over the wounds of a divorce.

If a divorcee leaps into an affair with a man immediately after her divorce, or into a second marriage, all she's doing is trying to cover up her lack of self-assurance. Marrying again on the rebound is notorious for repeating the mistakes of the failed marriage.

No. What you want—and are going to get—is something solid and lasting in the way of a relationship. That's why you are urged to build up your own self-esteem before letting another man come into your life. Note the phrase "letting a man come into your life." Not "looking for a man." Going where they are, yes. You can't catch fish in a rain barrel, and you have to be out there to be noticed.

Let a man see how special you are. You don't have to fling yourself at his head. If you're there, and exuding charm and self-confidence—*not* bereavement or loneliness—make no mistake, some man will notice you.

I remember one girl who was terminating an entanglement with a man she had thought of marrying. The longer she knew him, the less she thought of the whole idea. Most regretfully, because her love for him had been deep and sincere, she realized he had characteristics that would make a permanent relationship impossible. She saw less and less of him, although it hurt her.

Part of her job involved research in the public library. She became friendly with a librarian who was himself breaking off an unhappy relationship. No, they didn't wind up with a blazing romance. They were companions, however, for quite some time. Although each was open with the other about their past loves, there was nothing maudlin in their attitude. They had a happy friendship, then went on to something and someone else.

Each phase of life is different and should be taken at its own value. The dreams we had when we were young, the promise and magic of first love, are experiences never to be repeated. But the wonder and glory and plain fun of life is that every day, every hour, brings a new experience. It is responding to the challenge to make something new and whole out of something that seemed old, done with, shattered, that gives life a rich texture.

If you're widowed or divorced, you have a lot of experience to bring to any new relationship. Use it. Right here we get into the sticky question: How far should I go with a man?

That is entirely up to you. To go to bed with a man out of a sense of frustration or anger or because "I ought to," or "I miss sexual relations," is self-defeating. Don't think that a man who's any kind of man wants just a casual night with you. Any man who has known real sexual happiness may settle for something less—but it's always less. Sexual expertise is desirable, but anyone, man or woman, who has known fulfilling, lasting love knows how empty a mere sexual performance is.

Single girls also have to make their own choices. Again, what are you looking for? If it's just experience, that's what you'll get. You may or may not be able to use the experience later in cementing a permanent union—if a permanent union later on is what you want. I think it's fine that in these times—although marriage is, as far as I am concerned, the best way of living together—no one rejects the girl who elects to live otherwise.

Then there is the question often raised by single women: "Should I share an apartment to cut down expenses and avoid being lonely?" My personal reaction is that this is a mistake. You tend to narrow your social horizons this way. I knew some young mothers of young children who thought it would be a good, workable idea to share a house, thereby lightening the baby-sitting worries of those who had dates or jobs or outside interests, and lightening the housekeeping and other chores. With all the goodwill in the world, the experiment turned into a disaster. The children inevitably had little childish set-tos and couldn't be taken home to cool off—they *were* home. Every woman inevitably and naturally thinks her way of keeping house is best; these women found out the meaning of the old adage, "two women can't share the same kitchen." Not that they were openly critical, because they were really lovely, civilized women. But underneath, there was the yearning of each woman for her own little nest. Eventually, to save their sanity and their friendship, the group broke up.

Of course, there are women who do share a household, but it's not too often that it works out happily. Very young girls often share living quarters—but then, for very young girls it's an impermanent arrangement. Sooner or later they are going to find some young man, and off they'll go.

You, as a more mature woman, have to get back to the basics of being self-sufficient. You have an independent life to lead. Of course, if you find the man you'd like to take you away from all that, you will subtly let him know that he's the special one who can persuade you to give up your single blessedness.

Now, for women with small children: Don't think of your children as burdensome responsibilities that will keep you from having another man in your life. This isn't meant to sound callous or heartless—but has it occurred to you that you can use your children to find him? You can.

For instance, there are groups such as Parents Without Partners. A man who is concerned enough about his children to come to a group like this for help with his problems as a father is a man you're going to want to know better. He feels the way you do. Get to know each other, swap parent stories and problems and helpful discoveries—and who knows what may happen from there on?

There are school encounters. The longest journey, as the Chinese say, begins with but a single step, and from the time your children are in nursery school, you are stepping out with them into a world of new acquaintances, meetings, opportunities to get to know other parents, other children, other people. It's positively true that you can grow along with your children. In your case, not being wrapped up in their father, you will be free to notice other men. In the school systems, private and public, there are lots of them around.

One friend of mine mentioned with amusement that every time she took her niece to the park, wandered through the zoo, or rode with her on the carousel, more men noticed her than when she wandered through the park or the zoo alone. Possibly they felt that she was more approachable, obviously being in a position to smile and go away without any fuss than if she had been alone. Or possibly she was all the more appealing for showing love and attachment to a small person who obviously had nothing material to give her in return. Such freely given affection carries its own message to the beholder.

Picking people up isn't very sensible, as a rule, but with a child as a buffer, you have a good chance to study any man who comes over to chat about the child. A gesture to a child is certainly an inoffensive way to get acquainted. And you, because you are not in the least desperate to make the acquaintance of a man, any man, can stand off coolly and appraise whether his interest is sincere or otherwise.

Any mutual interest, in fact, can be a perfectly natural and aboveboard ice-breaker. There is a chemistry that works between people who are truly interested in the same subject. People quite naturally talk to each other at, for instance, a picture gallery. Camera enthusiasts quite naturally discuss lenses, angles, shutter speeds and subjects. As for events like flower shows, auctions, block parties, fund-raising get-togethers, and committees for anything at all, they are peopleacquainters par excellence. Just bring along your fascinating self, not your drab or disillusioned or self-pitying self, and you will attract someone as sure as pollen attracts bees.

Do you know the old story about the little ant who worked hard and got precious little for his efforts? He scoured the neighborhood in which he lived for crumbs to bring home. It was a difficult living, because he could get only one crumb here, another there. Another ant, noticing his struggles, said, "Why do you struggle for crumbs here and there, when on the near corner is a bakery? You can get crumbs there without half trying!"

A first-rate bakery for finding interesting, bright, dynamic men is politics. You are surrounded by men who are actively pushing toward a goal. It's so easy to get involved in all this swirl of activity. Volunteer your services at the local political club. You'll be snapped up.

However, if you're going to do volunteer work, don't let yourself get sidetracked into the lesser, backstage jobs, like sorting and filing papers and mail. Get yourself out front where the action is. Volunteer your services for campaigning, making speeches, writing speeches, doing liaison work. If you've had experience as a secretary, volunteer to do secretarial work for the candidates. And don't, in any of your work, ever efface yourself. You'll have to work hard, because these people expect it of you. But never, never, simply be a hero-worshiper. You'll end up hero-worshiping for the next twenty years, while more sparkling volunteers walk off with all the desirable men.

If you must support yourself, see if you can't get training that will fit you for working with politicians. I don't mean civil service, either. Many career girls, including top executives, have started at the secretarial level. Skills such as typing and shorthand aren't that hard to learn. What is really important to train is your mind. Train your mind to think charm, to think ability, to think promotion.

A girl who might have seemed to have everything against her worked in a governor's office. She was well over thirty, six feet tall, had never been married, had let her doctoral thesis slip by unfinished, wasn't particularly pretty. She got thoroughly involved in the governor's Presidential campaign, in the course of which she got to know another of the governor's staff. And eventually Nancy Maginnes married Secretary of State Henry Kissinger!

Most of all, you have to think of yourself as having some very special qualities to offer. Mature women have the advantage over young girls of having lived with themselves, gotten to know who they are. Young people are fresh and lovely, that's true, but they're also searching. Their forays out into life in search of adventure are really testings of themselves. What am I capable of? What has the world to offer me—and what price will I have to pay? Often enough, they're not aware of that latter part of the question.

You are. As the saying goes, you have been there and back. You are experienced in handling relationships. Even the divorcee, who has had to face the failure of a relationship, has learned many things from her experience. She has learned that men have needs and desires which may be, to her, irrational, but they are part of the masculine picture. She has also found out her own weaknesses. With age and experience there comes a priceless mellowing, an ability to look at a person's faults and still value that person as a whole. If you think a man doesn't prize this tolerance and accommodation, think again.

This graciousness, which can only be attained by living to what the French call *un certain âge*, can open doors for you if you yourself learn to value it. An experienced woman knows, thinks, responds with the intelligent awareness possible only to a woman who has experienced life as it really is.

Keep in mind that it is to be expected that you will have taken good care of your looks all this time! If for any reason you have neglected yourself, start this instant to give yourself all the pampering you should have.

I have deliberately left to the last the most important consideration of all. Your mental-emotional attitude will carry you to whatever life you are going to live from now on. It's perfectly true that what happens to you is not half so important as how you respond to what the fates have brought you. That same attitude will have an effect on what the fates will bring you next.

Consider this: If you have a mental picture of yourself as tired, frustrated, defeated, you will project that image, no matter how skillfully you try to hide it. You will attract to yourself only experiences that will carry out that unhappy mental image of what your life should be like.

Psychology comes in many schools, but there is one point on which all agree: Conditioning has much to do with how our later lives shape up; it is part of the story of how we use our minds. If you were conditioned as a little girl to think of yourself as pretty, vital and attractive, your mind will still project this image, and the image will reach other people's eyes: *pretty, vital, attractive*. People will see beyond any defect, and you will continue to act, from your inner conviction, as you always have. But even if our early conditioning has been negative, we must make every effort to feel deep within ourselves that we are worthwhile and that life still holds promise of pleasures and joys.

Let your inner conviction tell you that you have failed, that you are a grieving widow for whom life can never again be sweet, that you are doomed to dragging out your days alone and unfulfilled, and be you ever so outwardly bright and sparkling, you will unconsciously register drabness, defeat, emptiness. I don't know anyone outside a dedicated social worker who will want to have anything to do with such a person.

It is easier to say, Get over your griefs, than to do it. No one can really "get over" a private sorrow simply by willing it. The mind, the emotions, the psyche, have to adjust and readjust. The "gay divorcee" stereotype is someone who is trying to cover up her bitterness; the unflinching widow has tears to shed in secret; the defiant single girl who doesn't really like being single spends a lot of energy convincing herself as well as others that she really doesn't care.

What has to happen is that your mental energy must be refocused. This is where you have to practice being very, very kind to yourself. Acknowledge the sorrow that you have. Get it out in the open. One fundamental value of psychoanalysis is that you have the chance to get your old, unhealed regrets out into the open, to realize that you are not the horrible person that you thought you were. Or, conversely, that you're not really such a sweet, put-upon, blameless spiritual angel to whom everybody else is so unfeelingly rotten.

Yes, you have lost a loved husband. Yes, you made a terrible mess of your life: you chose the wrong man to marry; or you didn't do as much as you could have to save your marriage. Yes, you gave the best years of your life to coddling a mother who didn't love you anyway.

Now you have a choice. You can either stay with that terrible, gloomy condition. You can relive, over and over again, the misery and shock and pain you have known. Or you can put it all behind you—although it can never altogether leave your memory—and devote yourself to making tomorrow better than today.

You can't do this by willpower alone. We know now how the mind and emotions influence our subconscious reactions, how the subconscious influence on mind and emotion keeps us going around in an ever-narrowing circle, so that often we can't see anything except in the terms we have set for ourselves. I don't know how many women have been unable to see the true devotion some man was offering them, because they were imprisoned in an old, worn-out but still hurtful experience.

The only way you can free yourself from this web is via your imagination. I certainly don't mean that you should live in your dreams. But the magic of imagination is that, if you want to badly enough—and it must be you who wants it; no one else can do this for you—you can picture yourself as being different from what you are now. You can put the imagination to work with your subconscious and thereby create a new, happy self.

There are techniques for this. Whatever you are now is the result of the picture you have carried around, without realizing it, for a long time. Now that you have taken a long look at yourself, you see what it is you want to change. Then you picture the change as already accomplished. Then you tell your subconscious that you want it to have this new picture of you to project. And, if you really mean it, the subconscious effortlessly does this.

There's nothing mystical about any of this. It works in analysis, it works in religion, it will work for you.

This is one way you do it: Before you fall asleep, you are in a half-world, pulled away from all the busy thoughts that cluster around in your mind. You are relaxed, you are receptive to the thoughts that rise from your subconscious. Haven't you ever experienced sudden insights, or had marvelous ideas, just before you fell asleep? Now you talk to your inner self. You present the picture to your inner self of acting and being the way you want to act and be from now on. If you are firmly convinced of what you want, your inner self will take the suggestion and act upon it while you sleep. In days or weeks, depending on how firmly you have formed your belief, you will find yourself not only acting, but being, that new person.

This is not hocus-pocus. With all that science is exploring about our mental life, there is more and more proof that thought of this nature plays a larger role in our actions than was ever thought possible before.

Most of the time this sort of thing is going on anyway, without our being aware of it. Everything we do, every day, goes to form or reinforce or destroy the mental pictures we have of ourselves.

If you can't think beyond being a drudge, is it surprising if you remain one all your life? If you have the daring and vision to see yourself as being happily engaged in, say, scientific research, is it any wonder that you will make every effort to become a scientist, overcome obstacles because they aren't important in sight of your goal, and discover something that will benefit the world? The little girl who *solidly and firmly* sees herself as golf champion of the world works to attain her goal, and grows up to carry off the trophy.

You're no longer a child, you're a woman with a lot of experience behind you. You've undoubtedly failed at many things. But you've succeeded at a lot of things, too. That's where you have to put your thoughts. Remember how it felt; relive your emotions at that time. Think of that successful you, get into the habit of being that woman. Do things as if you were that woman again.

It really doesn't matter where you start. Just start. Fill your mind with all the positive things you can do. You can still go out and look at the roses. You can still go to the theater or a concert or even enjoy—but really enjoy—old movies on TV. You must exercise your mind, keep it active, just as you do your body. Or your mind will wither, exactly as your muscles will if you don't use them.

You can feel *alive*, all your life, with an active, inquiring, positive mind. Let it lead you into new, unfamiliar paths. If yesterday was good, cherish the memories and be thankful you have that much. (Some people, alas, don't.) If the past was terrible, you and you alone can build a better today. That's not a platitude; it's the solid truth.

I've said it before and I'll say it again: A truly attractive woman has an alive, inquiring mind. Even if your mental attitude right now is gloomy, with practice you can transpose the darkness into light. Without your bright mind, without the goal you set for yourself, nothing that happens to you from the outside will really change your life for the better.

You deserve the very best life has to offer. But changing your mental attitude is step number one. Then you'll find it both easy and profitable to follow all the other suggestions in this chapter. When they work to bring about a marvelous, fruitful life, don't be in the least surprised! Now go ahead, and do it.

11

Self-Awareness

Why is it that some women are always in the thick of things? They not only look their best; they seem to be exciting and interesting at any age. I like to look at faces of people in restaurants. Some people eat their way through the meal and go home. Others chat animatedly, laugh, and linger because whatever they are saying to one another holds their interest. I often wonder what on earth fascinates them so—I wish, for the moment, I were part of the group. They seem to have a capacity for diversion and a vitality that the silent eaters lack. Life is certainly not passing them by.

What I'm really asking is: Which group do you belong to? Is life for you a passive passing of time? Or are you in the mainstream of what's going on around you . . . joining in it . . . enjoying it? Do you join in conversations? Is this you? In other words, Are you with it?

I've devised a little test for you to take. There are no winners or losers. It's a test designed to make you more aware of yourself and the world around you. It may be a shock to find out how time is passing you by; on the other hand, you may learn how much you are keeping up with the world around you and realize what a good time you're really having.

If you have come to the sorry realization that indeed you've slipped, not just physically, but in every way, then use this test as a catalyst for a change in your life. You need the world and the world needs you. Join it! Get with it!

1. What do you think of Bianca Jagger?

It doesn't matter what you think of Bianca Jagger; the point of the question is, Do you even know who she is? Bianca is the highly publicized wife of rock star Mick Jagger and is forever in the gossip columns and fashion magazines. She typifies no one; she is of the new wave of nonentities who receive much public attention, but if you don't know who she is you're not keeping up with the "beautiful people." It's a frivolous pastime, but fun.

2. What new recipes have you tried lately?

If you haven't tried anything new for lunch or dinner, you're becoming set in your ways, and possibly boring whoever has to eat with you every day. Read *Gourmet* or some other magazine devoted to cooking, and don't just read: Try something new every week.

3. What books have you read lately?

I hope you've read lots, both fiction and nonfiction. Books give you ideas, and ideas are what are needed to keep your mind active.

4. Do you read the financial pages in the newspaper?

If you don't read this important section of the paper, you can't really know what's going on in your own life, as the financial world affects you in many ways. Also, men love to talk finance, and you're left out of many conversations if you can't at least listen intelligently.

5. What do you see in a fashion magazine?

If you merely look at the pictures, then put the magazine down, you're missing the point of the whole thing. You don't have to buy the clothes you see there, but read the copy for what's new. Adapt the fashions of the times for your own use.

Study the makeup, the hair, and then think about how you can incorporate these new trends into your own life.

6. Do you know the name of your state and national Congressmen and Senators?

If you don't, then I can assume you're not very interested in today's issues. These deeply affect our lives; and you should be writing to your government representatives expressing your opinions. This is one of the ways you can actively participate in government without really working in it.

7. Have you tried TM?

Transcendental meditation seems to be sweeping the world. It's a form of relaxation vastly beneficial to many people. For people who drink to excess, who are on drugs, or are hypertense, TM seems to be an enormous help. I tried it, but find that I get more from yoga. It's really worth investigating.

8. What is a Cuisinart?

Aha! If you don't know, you don't like to cook much. A Cuisinart is like having another pair of hands in the kitchen. It chops, shreds and does everything but put the food on the stove. It is a very expensive gadget, but worth it.

9. Who are the star pitchers and quarterbacks of your local baseball and football teams?

You should know and keep up with sports unless you are married to or going with that rare male who doesn't like them. In any case, not knowing about golf, swimming, hockey, baseball, basketball, and football leaves you out of many conversations.

10. Who are the heads of goverment of France, Germany, England, Italy, Russia, India, China, Egypt, and Israel?

These are not the only nations in the world, but they play a large part in shaping our lives today and tomorrow. Your awareness of the world is in large part indicated by what you know about these influential leaders.

11. Have you changed your eyeglass frames lately?

Next time you change the prescription, change the frame. I never knew until I changed mine what a difference a new frame can make in one's appearance.

12. Do you ever change the decor of your home?

Do you add or move pictures, change colors, reupholster? Even a new shade or curtain can add a new dimension to a room. Liven things up with new plants and flowers for a new look.

13. Do you clean out your closet and discard clothes and "things" that you are not wearing or using?

Getting rid of unused clothes and odds and ends clears out the clutter and frees you for something new. Don't keep saying, I might need these some day. You won't.

14. Do you have plans for future projects and work toward them?

I hope so, because if you only live for today, you're really in a rut. Even if you only dream about going to the Antarctic, or living someplace else, dreams are what life is made of, and you should have some.

15. Have you read a serious book about sexual enjoyment?

If you haven't, you may be missing something in your life.

16. Have you taken a course in anything lately?

I don't care if it's gardening, Chinese cooking, knitting, French or economics. All local high schools offer a variety of adult education courses. They keep you interested, not bored —and interested is what you should be.

17. When did you last buy yourself some pretty lingerie?

If you neglect the little feminine things in life, you'll be neglected.

18. Do you read a variety of magazines?

You should try to glean the best from a variety of magazines. News, theater, gardening, fashion, beauty, homemaking, politics, medicine, the world is there for you to know about . . . talk about.

I could ask you questions ad infinitum, but as I complete the last one, I realize that what I'm trying to say is, It's all a question of attitude. Think about the facets of your life—your family relationships, friends; your face, hair and body; your home. The whole person is the sum of many parts. Examine each aspect of your life; and if something is missing, find and develop it—for then and only then can you live life to its fullest.

12

Women Speak for Themselves

When I was preparing this book, I decided to make up a questionnaire designed to find out how women *really* live, what they expect from life, what disappointments have come their way. To get a wide range of experiences and opinions, I mailed batches of the questionnaires to friends all over the country, asking them to send them on to individual friends, or to names picked at random out of the telephone book. The questionnaires were sent out anonymously, and all the recipients were assured that I would have no way of knowing who they were. No names or addresses were asked for; one simply had to fill out the questionnaire and mail it back to me at the agency.

The survey, as you'll be able to see from the answers printed here, really cut across a wide spectrum of both age and income. That makes our primary finding all the more extraordinary, I think. Because by and large, the great majority of women who answered are happy with the lives they've made for themselves.

Here's how it breaks down.

Of all the women who responded to the survey, a huge 77 percent answered that, yes, they considered themselves happily married. That left only 23 percent answering negatively.

That's a tremendous response, especially when you consider how many people are proclaiming the demise of marriage as an institution. As we get further into the survey's specific questions, you'll be able to see exactly where the problems and dissatisfactions do arise. However, the fact that more than 75 percent of the women answered that on the whole they were happy in their marriages, is to me a very encouraging statistic. Almost all said if marriage were a renewable contract, they would renew!

And most of these marriages have lasted a pretty long time! Only 5% of the respondents had been married for a year or less; 71% were married for between one and twenty-five years, and a full 24 percent, or almost exactly one fourth of the women, had been married for more than twenty-five years!

The questionnaire reached a very wide range of incomes as well. Half the incomes were below $25,000 and half were above. The lower half broke down this way: 19 percent had earnings for the family of below $15,000 and 32 percent had earnings of between $15,000 and $20,000. The upper half had 24 percent in the $25,000-to-$50,000 bracket, and 25 percent reported incomes of over $50,000 per year.

Here's the way the percentages broke down according to age group:

18–25	2%
25–30	28%
30–40	42%
40–50	12%
over 50	16%

Then we got to the specific questions about what women like and dislike about their husbands. First, personality considerations.

Seventy-seven percent find their mates mentally stimulating. Their reasons were primarily that he was intelligent/well-informed (27 percent) and had an interesting background

(20 percent). His interests, said 20 percent, and ability to converse (15 percent), followed by his sense of humor and the work he did (each of the latter cited by 12 percent of the respondents), made husbands good companions.

When I asked what personality traits the respondents would like to see changed in their husbands, a big 58 percent preferred no changes at all! Those who did want to see what they felt would be an improvement in the personality of their men were almost evenly divided into groups concerned with temper, jealousy, lack of understanding, lack of communication. Between 4 percent and 6 percent mentioned such characteristics.

By far the largest number of wives (71 percent) declared that their husbands' mental attitudes fell between good and excellent. A fourth of the women thought them to be changeable, depressed, or stuck in the attitudes of their early upbringing, and thus out of step with today's world. But only 2% found that last category to be descriptive of their husbands.

I asked blunt questions about the physical appearance of the husbands and about the couples' sexual relations.

Although 53 percent wouldn't make any change (even if change were possible), women complained about loss of hair and added poundage in equal numbers, 11 percent expressing disappointment in their men in these areas. About 7 percent wished their husbands would show better taste in selecting their clothes, and forty-four percent wished the men would take better care of themselves. Among the miscellaneous complaints voiced by a few, I'm afraid there's nothing I can recommend for the women who wished their husbands were taller!

An overwhelming 98 percent of the women answering the survey thought that their husbands had aged well. An equal number replied that skin condition was good, although a slightly smaller number (93 percent) said that body condition was all it should be. The figure dropped to 88 percent when I asked whether they approved of his hair style.

Yet with all these good marks in hubby's favor, 40 percent

found that other men were more attractive (maybe they were thinking of Paul Newman). Forty-four percent wished that their men would take better care of themselves. But when we asked that the husbands be rated on a scale from one to ten on such items as sex appeal, personality, and awareness, most wives gave their husbands a score of nine!

Then we got into questions relating to sex. A lucky 91 percent still found their husbands sexually appealing. The 9 percent who did not divided their reasons evenly between the following factors: lack of affection on the husband's part; selfishness that made him insensitive to the needs of his wife; and lack of sexual freedom because of subjection to the inhibitions of the fifties.

Eighty-nine percent of the women indicated that they would not want any change in their sex relations with their husbands. The remaining 11 percent opted for greater frequency. One woman penciled in that the one thing she would like to change in her sex life was "forgetting all that my mother told me, and the taboos that I was brought up with."

A number of the women who wanted to increase the frequency of their sex relations fell into the eighteen-to-twenty-five age group, while most of the forty-to-fifty-and-over groups told me that they liked things just fine the way they are!

Yet, when we totaled up the categories that provided most of the mutual interest between husband and wife, sex came out low on the totem pole, with only 5 percent indicating that this was the area where they found most common ground. The areas of more importance were:

Sports	29%
Children	20%
Travel	13%
Working together	10%
Friends	8%

These were the preferences of the additional 80 percent who expressed having mutual interests. Of the 15 percent who replied that they had none, 2 percent mentioned football as the culprit; one woman said her husband was interested in nothing else but, and furthermore did not think it necessary that women have any interests at all.

Interestingly, the same figures of 85 percent and 15 percent crop up when I asked about being bored with life in general. Again, the larger group had the more positive answer, while the same percentage of women who said they had no mutual interests in common with their husbands (15 percent) were also bored with their lives. The reasons given for this boredom was very evenly spread out, the causes given as lack of purpose, lack of activity, lack of friends, desire for independence, dislike for tasks, and the "housewife syndrome."

We also asked about children. Twenty-nine percent didn't have any; of those who did, the ages ranged from infancy to twenty-five years and over. No family had more than four.

One of the most interesting aspects of the survey was the fact that to the first question, "Are you married?" 15 percent of the respondents said no, and then went on to answer *all* the husband-and-wife questions, with varying responses. Obviously they were all in one sort of housekeeping situation or other. Many had children. All seemed to consider their partners the same as if they were married. And this situation cut across *all* age groups. Maybe the kids living together these days haven't started something so new after all!

Another interesting aspect of the survey has to do with drinking habits. We hear so much these days about the alarmingly increasing rate of alcoholism—in fact, it was my concern about this problem that led me to include these questions in my survey. I wanted to find out how much drinking American women were actually doing, and why.

The answers again were a surprise, and again the surprise was on the pleasant side.

Although 80 percent of the respondents said that they drank, only 8 percent drank a lot. Eleven percent drank only in social situations, 14 percent at mealtimes (I hope they will read my chapters on drinking and dieting), 28 percent drank moderately, and 39 percent, the largest group, drank very little.

Among the women who admitted to being depressed (11 percent as against 89 percent who are not), 22 percent could give no reason. The others were, again, very evenly divided as to the causes of their depression. About the same percentage of women answered yes to each of these reasons: finances, children, fatigue from work, unrealized ambitions, the strain of family life, and life in general.

Only 13 percent of the women answered that they are nervous. Of these, 25 percent considered themselves to be hyperactive, while the causes for nervousness cited by the remainder all had to do with pressure in one form or another. Pressures of business and financial problems, difficulty in meeting goals and fulfilling material wants accounted for the increasing nervousness of these individuals. It would seem that the more that women go out into the world, the more such problems seem to extract their toll. That fact seems inescapable. In a related question, I asked how many were in actual fear of losing their mates and only 9 percent answered that this was indeed the case. Most of the nervousness reported does not seem to stem from the marital relationship itself, but rather from other, outside pressures. Only 7 percent of those who were afraid of losing their husbands were seeing marriage counselors; the fear, for those 50 percent who were increasing their attempts to please their husbands and the 43 percent who were trying to improve their appearance, may indeed have been more imaginary than real. In any case, trying harder to work at one's marriage is in itself a positive step that can prevent problems before they start. And I'm all for that!

There you have it: a cross section of American women looking at their lives, their husbands, and themselves. On the whole, I am very pleased with the results of my research. However I do see that there are indications that may be danger signals. While the institution of marriage seems to be in much better working order than anyone dared hope for, there are still problems and uncertainties that face more and more women, and these may be increasing. After all, the more one sees of the world, the more one sees of its problems, and the more those problems add to one's own.

I don't take this in any way to mean that women should stop the marvelous progress that they have made in every area of endeavor. What the survey did for me, in analyzing all those was to point out that there are indeed dangers in this new-found freedom, and that we must recognize this fact. Let us not for a moment think that the woman who confines herself solely to husband, house, and family is not going to have any troubles. The problems of the "housewife syndrome" may be even more extreme than they are for the woman who has developed outlets that channel more of her brains and energy. New circumstances always bring new problems; the important thing is to be aware of and to anticipate these problems.

Conducting this survey gave me the feeling that I was indeed in contact with many women. It was a great help in formulating the subjects I wanted to discuss with you. Now that the book is just about finished, I feel very strongly that I would like to continue the communication. I invite your letters, not only to tell me what you think of the book (so many readers are so lovely in the tributes that they send in and no writer is immune to them!!) but to continue the dialogue. Let me know how my vegetarian diet worked for you—how many pounds lost, how many inches you've pared away. As good friends and neighbors have always done, I'd like to exchange recipes with you. I've given you *my* low-calorie favorites; how about giving me some of yours?

Or perhaps you'd like to add your own statistics to the survey. Let me know your personal reaction to some of the questions. I feel that all of life is a continuing process, each part closely linked to those that preceded it and those that will follow it as well. I would like the exchange of information initiated here to have that kind of continuum, too. Just as my experiences and those of others helped form my earlier books, so perhaps will the new things you tell me become part of another book.

With the women of middle years who answered my questionnaire I share a common bond of faith—faith in our ability to make these years a good and worthwhile time in our lives. To those who, like me, have at times given in to the pressures that seemed unbearable and the obstacles that seemed insurmountable, I can only reemphasize what I have stated throughout this book—that there is never a time too early nor a time too late to begin the business of living—to improve what needs improving in ourselves and in our lives. To change an attitude or reshape a figure is well within the power of each of us. All of the plans and suggestions I've described here can work for you. It's up to you to take what I've told you to heart and to incorporate all these ideas into your daily life so that you can reap the full benefit. I say "reap" for a reason. Reading a book like this is something like planting seeds. The promise is there, but the work has to be done. Only then can you see and pick the beautiful flowers, the bouquet of life that is yours to enjoy forever. I know—I did it.

If what I've written so far has not inspired you, the following pages could be the most important pages you've looked at in a long time. Here are photographs of some of the world's greatest models, as lovely today as they were ten, twenty, thirty and forty years ago! Mothers, grandmothers, career women— all a living testament to the fact that care makes the difference. Most did not conceal their age.

These women know who and what they were and are. They are confident. Those years of self-discipline as famous beauties have served them well. Healthful diet, exercise, and wide-ranging interests have made them beautiful inside as well as out.

There is no reason why a woman of any age can not do the same thing. This is the point in life when you can change. There's no shame to admitting to yourself or those around you (if you want to) that you'd like to change your looks or life-style for the better. The only person who can do that is you! This is a message I've tried to get across to women at every opportunity. Why not take care of yourself? Most of us are too busy taking care of others; but part of taking care of others is taking care of yourself. Florence Dornan Formwalt wrote me that many of her daughter's teen-age friends had come to her for beauty advice over the years, because they didn't want to look like their mothers when they grew up. That says a great deal. Those close to you do observe and take pride in how you look. They can't have that pleasure if you don't make the effort yourself.

We are living in a different world. The prairie woman is preserved on television and in history books only. Youth and vigor can be maintained long past the time when these poor souls were in their graves. We can't hide in the past. The world is around us to meet head on.

The woman who says "It's too late" is, in a sense, burying herself! It is not too late, not for you nor anyone else. Look at the women on the following pages; some are much older than you. They prove that the world of beauty is not limited to the very young. It's a big wonderful world that can be shared by everyone; and by "everyone," I mean you!

13

*Former Models
Speak Up Today*

Jean Patchett Auer

1. *What years did you model?*
   1948–1960
2. *How many children do you have?*
   Two.
3. *Have you any grandchildren?*
   No.
4. *What were your weight and measurements as a model?*
   115–120 pounds; 34–24–35; 5 feet 9 inches.
5. *What are your weight and measurements today?*
   120–122 pounds. Decided I had better measure: 35–26½–35.
6. *Do you diet? If so, how?*
   No.
7. *How do you care for your skin?*
   Cleansing cream and astringent, night cream, hot and cold water.
8. *Do you exercise? If so, how often and how long?*
   Yes, in the morning, once a day—five minutes.
9. *How do you care for your hair?*

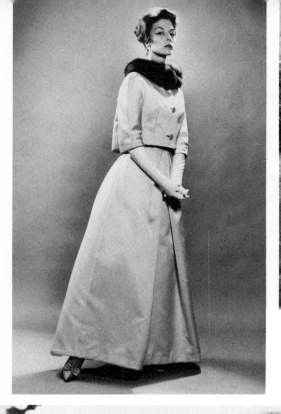
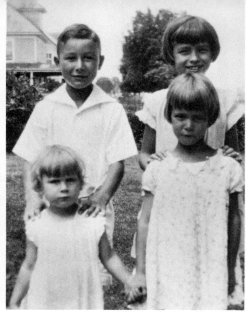
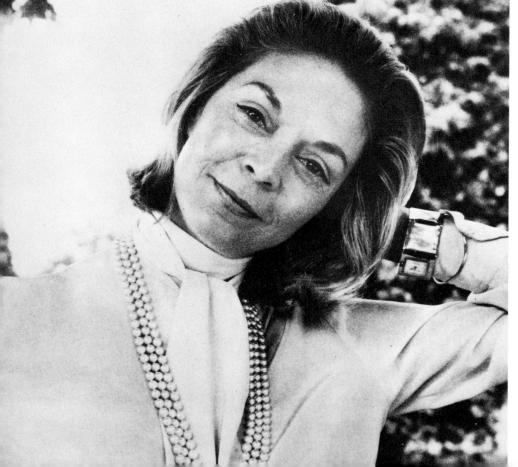

Wash it once a week and put it up every night. Brush it a great deal.

10. *What do you do to keep happy and interested in the world?*
    Taking care of my husband and children, playing bridge, doing needlepoint, working for my two charities, playing golf and taking tennis lessons, etcetera, etcetera, etcetera.

11. *Do you mind saying how old you are for publication?*
    Yes, I do mind.

12. *Do you have what you consider a coordinated beauty and/or health program?*
    Yes.

13. *Have you had or would you consider plastic surgery?*
    No, I have never had it. Yes, I would consider it.

14. *How do you feel about what is called "middle age"?*
    I suppose there is such a thing and I suppose I am in that age, but I sure don't feel like it or will I ever feel that I am in "middle age" or "old age." I think young.

Jane Cartwright Carlson

1. *What years did you model?*
   Since 1948—still going.
2. *How many children do you have?*
   Three sons—ages twenty-three, twenty, sixteen.
3. *Have you any grandchildren?*
   Not that I know of.
4. *What were your measurements as a model?*
   In the beginning, 33–22–33.
5. *What are your measurements today?*
   Now, 34–25–35 (spread a lot). I do not try to maintain same measurements as when I was twenty years old because I think the face looks drawn when you are older and too thin. And the face is more important.
6. *Do you diet? If so, how?*
   I do not diet as such; however, I am careful to eat the correct, balanced foods. Foods such as avocado, bananas, potatoes are high in calories but very nutritious, and I eat tons. Never touch pastry and only whole-grain bread— lots of fruit, salad, and no fats and gravies and desserts.

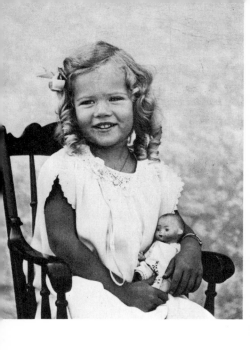
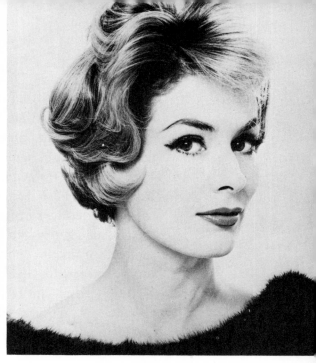
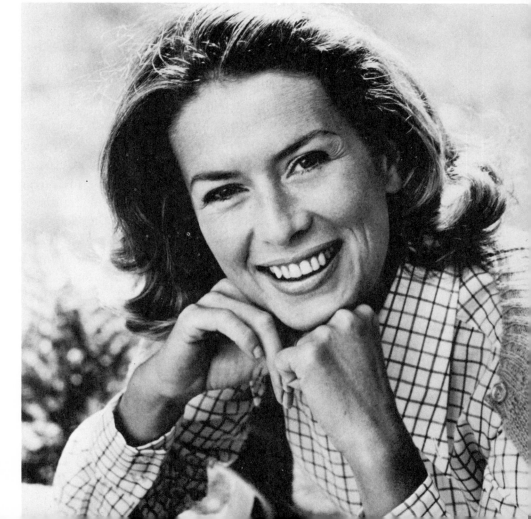

7. *How do you care for your skin?*

Cleanse well with a cleansing cream, wash with a pure soap (Oilatum) and rinse till skin "squeaks," then liberal dose of moisturizer before retiring and under makeup.

8. *Do you exercise? If so, how often and how long?*

My facial skin has held well because my weight never changes radically, so there hasn't been any stretching. I exercise moderately—walking and bicycling, swimming in summer. Again, not enough, but am a very active person.

9. *How do you care for your hair?*

Nothing special—am fortunate not to have any gray and also my hair isn't oily. All I do is treat it well, brush, and add a lotion to give it body before setting.

10. *What do you do to keep happy in the world?*

I am a professional painter and have had this interest even before modeling. I think another interest or hobby is totally important for a model as a stabilizer. Otherwise your physical self becomes *too* important, and when the looks begin to fade the morale goes with them. I have always looked at modeling as a lovely "frosting on the cake"—to be taken seriously and professionally, not however to let it become one's sole purpose in life. Now, as I have more time away from the world of fashion, I paint every spare minute, and am gradually moving my career into the world of art. It can be a very smooth transition and almost as financially rewarding. Many models have made this sort of transition into another pursuit. Also, I've found the art to have been a help to my modeling. I am always thinking design, shape and composition from the camera's point of view.

11. *Do you mind saying how old you are for publication?*

No. I am forty-four. I tell it because now it is an asset. There is loads of work for my age group, and to try to be anything but what you are is only fooling yourself.

12. *Do you have what you consider a coordinated beauty and/or health program?*

I do think past training as a model *makes* you form good habits—you never let up. I know my husband is grateful when he looks at me, and I *care* what he thinks.

13. *Have you had or would you consider plastic surgery?*
    I have not had any, but see nothing wrong with it for a real problem, such as "bags," pouches, jowls, etcetera—but not for the purpose of making a fifty-year-old into a twenty-year-old. It doesn't work anyway; everyone looks the same—slanty-eyed.

14. *How do you feel about what is called "middle age"?*
    I love it. I'm happy. I know how to live, what I like, and where I'm going. I think you accept life and are not in such a big rush to nowhere.

Suzy Parker Dillman

1. *What years did you model?*

   From the age of fourteen, which would have been the summer of 1947, since I was born October 28, 1932. I retired when I became pregnant with the first child of my marriage to Bradford Dillman (we married April 19, 1963), and that would have been the spring of 1965 when I was thirty-two. During those eighteen years I also worked as a fashion photographer for the French Vogue and I acted in movies and T.V.

2. *How many children do you have?*

   Four of my own and two stepchildren whom I consider as my own. My oldest daughter, Georgia De La Salle, is just sixteen, Dinah Dillman is ten, Charles Dillman is eight, and Christopher Dillman is seven. My stepchildren are Pamela Dillman, sixteen, and Jeffrey Dillman, eighteen, who has just been accepted at Duke University for this fall.

3. *Have you any grandchildren?*

   Not for at least ten years, please God.

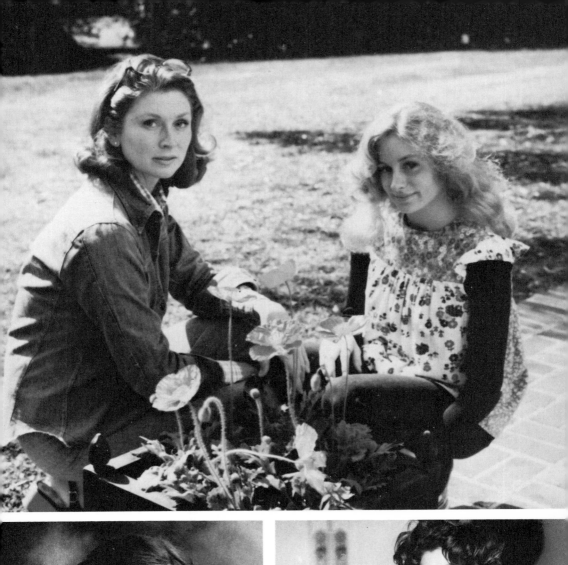

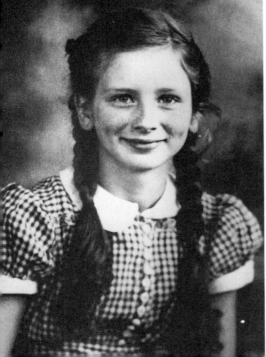

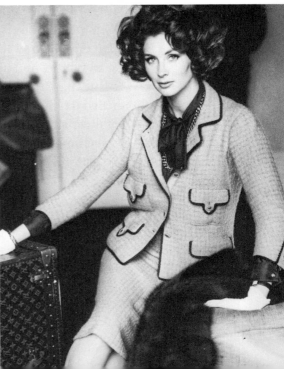

4. *What were your weight and measurements as a model?*
Over the years from 115 pounds to 135. I'm 5 feet 9 inches tall. For most of my career as a model I was a size ten to twelve.

5. *What are your measurements today?*
I weigh 134 and I'm still a ten to twelve, and still wearing all my old Chanel suits.

6. *Do you diet? If so, how?*
I eat less of everything—no desserts.

7. *How do you care for your skin?*
I have used Erno Laszlo's products for twenty years. He was my dermatologist. It's basically putting oil on my face before I soap it and never leaving cream on my face at night. It's also nicer for my husband to sleep with a lady who does not look greased to swim the English Channel!

8. *Do you exercise? If so, how often and how long?*
I swim almost every day. I do laps in an outdoor Olympic-sized pool at the Biltmore Hotel. It's fortunate that in Santa Barbara the weather is almost always great!

9. *How do you care for your hair?*
Shabbily, but fortunately I've always had good strong hair. I have never used dyes or hair colors. I now have a few white hairs among the red and I directly attribute them to my two teen-aged girls.

10. *What do you do to keep happy and interested in the world?*
I read politics and history. Literature is my passion. I love to garden, particularly with roses. I'm a pretty good gourmet cook. I have a wonderful husband, whose talent as an actor delights me. I adore my children.

11. *Do you mind saying how old you are for publication?*
I enjoy being my age, forty-four.

12. *Do you have what you consider a coordinated beauty and/or health program?*
I use the Laszlo products, I swim every day. That's it.

13. *Have you had or would you consider plastic surgery?*
    I do not believe in plastic surgery for cosmetic purposes. I believe in Coco Chanel's definition of beauty: "A woman can only be judged beautiful after she's forty, for then she has the face she deserves."
14. *How do you feel about what is called "middle age"?*
    It's great to be alive. I enjoy watching the growth of my children and their evolvement. My marriage is more beautiful because of our maturity and the length of our friendship.

    P.S. I feel it most important to credit my sister, Dorian Leigh, one of the most famous fashion models of all time, with my involvement in modeling, and eventual success.

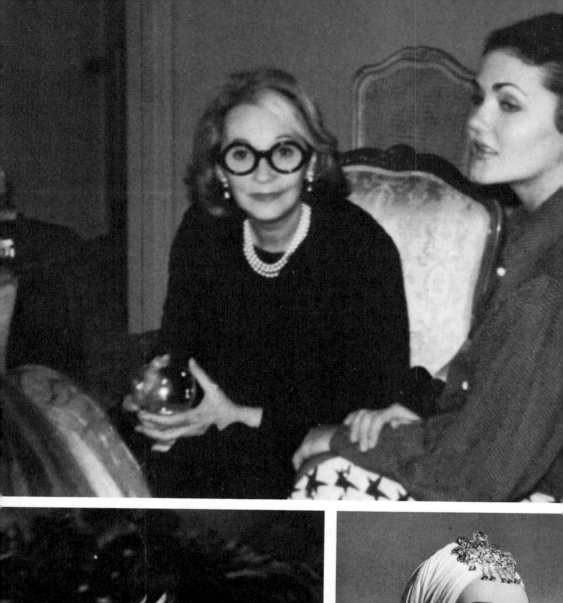
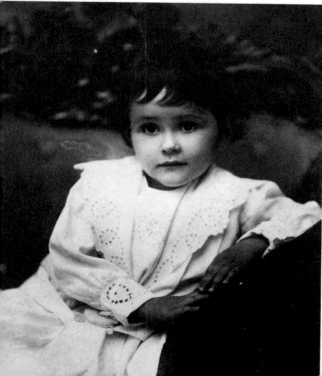
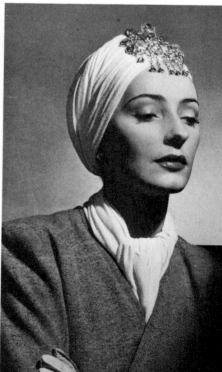

Betty Dorso

1. *What years did you model?*
   1929–1950'ish; in the fifties as a personality.
2. *How many children do you have?*
   Three.
3. *Have you any grandchildren?*
   Between us we have ten; six are mine.
4. *What were your weight and measurements as a model?*
   5 feet 9½ inches; 125 pounds; 34–24–34.
5. *What are your measurements today?*
   36–28–38; size ten to twelve.
6. *Do you diet? If so, how?*
   No sweets, starch.
7. *How do you care for your skin?*
   Inherited good skin. Once a week, soap. Pond's Cold Cream, others; Revanescence moisturizer under powders, cream at night.
8. *Do you exercise? If so, how often and how long?*
   Fifteen minutes every A.M. Walk a lot.

9. *How do you care for your hair?*
   Shampoo once a week, no coloring, set once a week, brush a lot.
10. *What do you do to keep happy and interested in the world?*
    Wake up at 6 A.M., in love with life, people, especially open-minded friends. We edit out anyone who is not mature in thought, whether young or old. Enjoy entertaining and cooking. Read constantly; love being home with my family. Our store is a joy.
11. *Do you mind saying how old you are for publication?*
    Born 1911. Sixty-six in October.
12. *Do you have what you consider a coordinated beauty and/or health program?*
    Feeling fit comes primarily from enjoying every moment and being "up."
13. *Have you had or would you consider plastic surgery?*
    Have not had, but would not hesitate if I thought necessary. Face is still good, could get rid of chin.
14. *How do you feel about what is called "middle age"?*
    Hard to answer, don't feel middle-aged. Too active.

Florence Formwalt

1. *What years did you model?*

   1939–1945, then spasmodically through 1950—when I worked six months for you.
2. *How many children do you have?*

   Three.
3. *Have you any grandchildren?*

   No.
4. *What were your weight and measurements as a model?*

   33½–22½–33½; 115 pounds.
5. *What are your measurements and weight today?*

   33½–23½–33½; 112 pounds.
6. *Do you diet? If so, how?*

   Not really. Some thirty-odd years ago I learned to enjoy what are now called natural foods. This, plus a diet high in protein and low in starch and fat has kept my weight within a five-pound range for twenty-five years.
7. *How do you care for your skin?*

   Basically, I try to keep it very clean, well lubricated, changing the treatment to suit the weather. In winter I use cleansing cream, liquid cleanser, along with moisturizer and night cream. In summer I use a fatted soap; sun screen, if I'm in the sun. I also take Vitamin E.

8. *Do you exercise? If so, how often and how long?*

Since I run a nursery, garden shop and landscaping service, life is very active physically during most of the year, and no additional exercise is needed. However, during the months of December through February, I do calesthenics about twenty minutes a day, followed by a short jog.

9. *What do you do to keep happy and interested in the world?*

I stay very interested in national and world affairs, have been the only woman on a town planning commission for three years, passionately adore movies, do landscape design as a profession and Japanese gardening and propagating more plants as a hobby. I design and make most of my own clothes, work for civic beautification through the Theman Society—and that's only the beginning.

10. *Do you mind saying how old you are for publication?*

No. I'm fifty-five. I used to mind, but both my girls started telling all their friends how old I was. When I asked them why, they said they did it because they were proud of me. That did it—now I don't care.

11. *Do you have what you consider a coordinated beauty and/or health program?*

Simplicity, moderation and basic rules of good health.

12. *How do you feel about what is called "middle age"?*

I think it's challenging. Each time you lose something you gain something, and can constantly adapt and accept the challenge. When I was very young someone told me, "There are four ages of woman: the age of beauty, the age of charm, the age of wit and the age of wisdom, and in each age, we must prepare for the next." If one tries to do this well, it is enough for a lifetime.

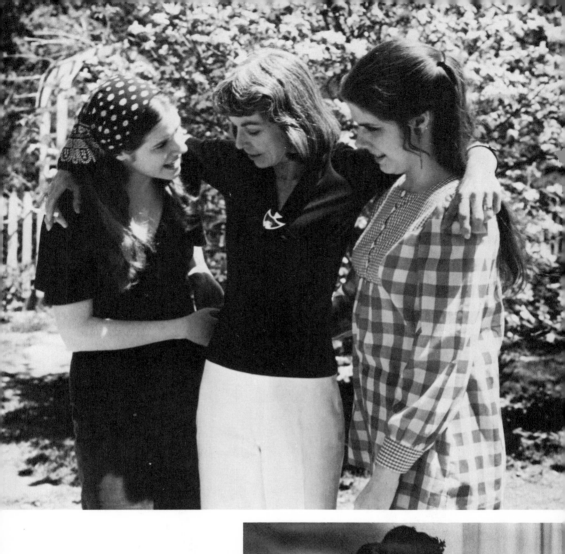

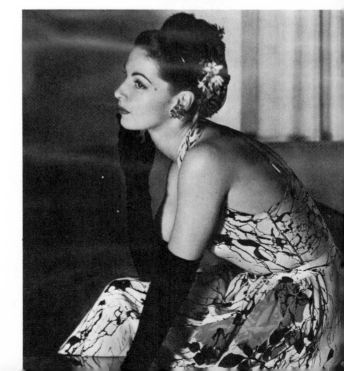

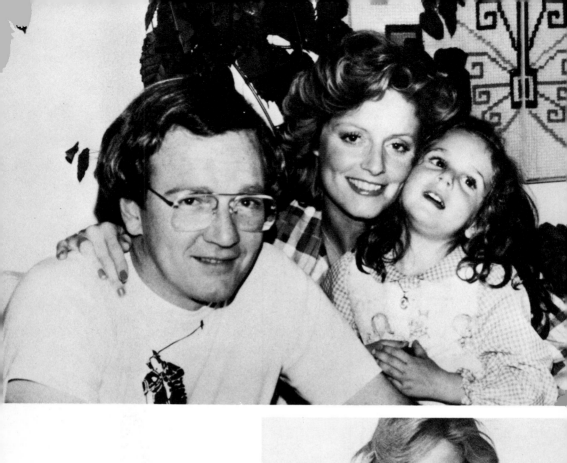

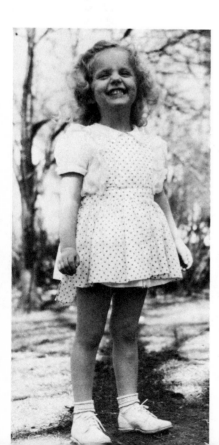

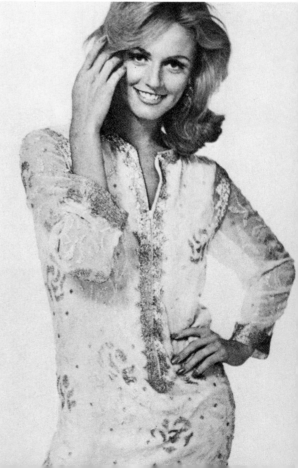

Sunny Griffin

1. *What years did you model?*
   1962–1975.
2. *What were your weight and measurements as a model?*
   5 feet 8 inches; 120 pounds; 34–24–35.
3. *What are your measurements today?*
   Same, normally, but now I'm pregnant.
4. *Do you diet? If so, how?*
   I make sure I get three well-balanced meals a day involving at least two servings of protein, three fresh vegetables, two kinds of fruit, some grain products—and now that I'm pregnant, a quart of skim milk. I try to avoid "empty calories."
5. *How do you care for your skin?*
   I use a cleanser and freshener twice a day and a very good moisturizer.
6. *Do you exercise? If so, how often and how long?*
   I think exercise is the most important thing you can do for yourself. I go to a gym three times a week (Kounovsky in New York City and Ron Fletcher in Los Angeles) and

play tennis daily when at home in Los Angeles. I also ski as much as possible.

7. *How do you care for your hair?*

My hair is naturally very curly and I cannot handle it, so I have it done professionally (just blown dry-straight) twice a week. I have it frosted about three or four times a year by Robert Renn in New York City.

8. *What do you do to keep happy and interested in the world?*

I work!! I am beauty editor for Avon, which involves a great deal of traveling around the country. I am fascinated by my husband's work as a CBS news correspondent and am constantly thrilled by our three-and-one-half-year-old daughter, Kelly, as we anxiously await our new arrival.

9. *Do you mind saying how old you are for publication?*

I am thirty-five and proud of it! Born November 17, 1940.

10. *Do you have what you consider a coordinated beauty and/or health program?*

I think a sensible diet, together with exercise and good grooming, is a terrific beauty program. Also, I don't smoke, drink very little, and hate staying up late.

11. *Have you had or would you consider plastic surgery?*

I would definitely consider plastic surgery.

12. *How do you feel about what is called "middle age"?*

"Middle age" is what you make of it. Some people are extremely old, others extremely young! I just want to look as good as Eileen Ford in a bikini at fifty!

Lillian Fox Groueff

1. *What years did you model?*
   1938–1941.
2. *How many children do you have?*
   Four.
3. *Have you any grandchildren?*
   Four.
4. *What were your weight and measurements as a model?*
   110 pounds; 32–21–35
5. *What are your measurements today?*
   120 pounds; 34–23–36
6. *Do you diet? If so, how?*
   No bread, sweets, liquor.
7. *How do you care for your skin?*
   Janet Sartin Salon products.
8. *Do you exercise? If so, how often and how long?*
   Skiing, tennis, bodyworks—three times a week, one hour.
9. *How do you care for your hair?*
   Wash at home. Cut at Cinandre and brush-dry. Brush-dry it myself in between.

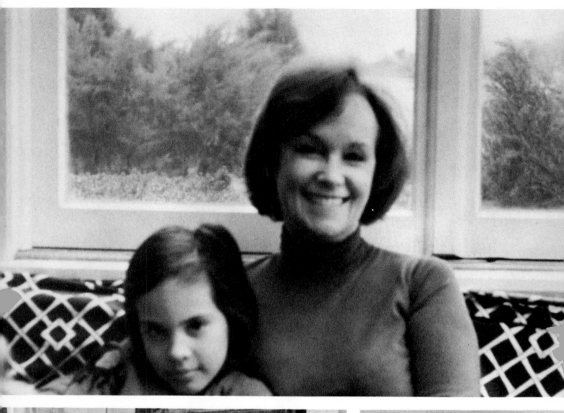

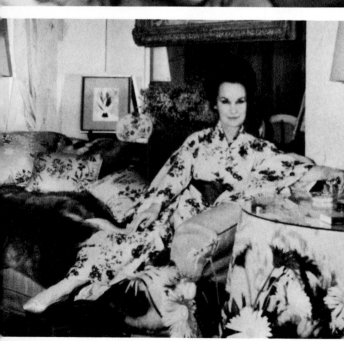

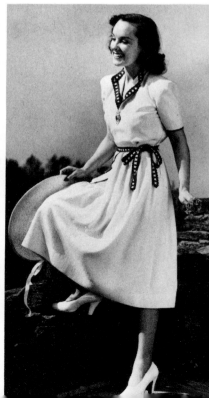

10. *What do you do to keep happy and interested in the world?*
    Interior design, painting, seeing my family, entertaining friends, traveling, discovering new things all the time.
11. *Do you mind saying how old you are for publication?*
    I don't tell myself ever.
12. *Do you have what you consider a coordinated beauty and/or health program?*
    Fairly so.
13. *Would you consider plastic surgery?*
    Yes.
14. *How do you feel about what is called "middle age"?*
    It is the same as middle spread. A healthy sex life probably helps to keep one healthy and young in spirit.

Sunny Harnett

1. *What years did you model?*
   Continuously from 1949 to 1962. Twelve years with Fords.
2. *How many children do you have?*
   One boy, Michael, now sixteen years old.
3. *Have you any grandchildren?*
   Not yet.
4. *What were your weight and measurements as a model?*
   5 feet 9½ inches; 114 pounds; 33–23–33.
5. *What are your weight and measurements today?*
   Pretty much the same.
6. *Do you diet? If so, how?*
   No.
7. *How do you care for your skin?*
   Very gently and every day. Cleansing, moisturizing, and makeup for the day.
8. *Do you exercise? If so, how often and how long?*
   Walking is the best and most natural exercise.

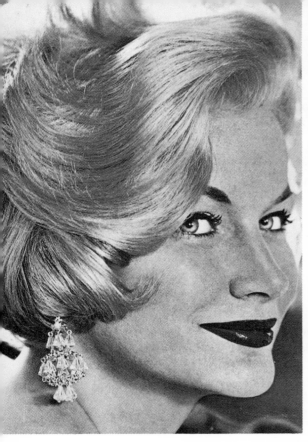

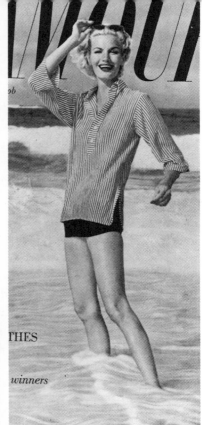

winners

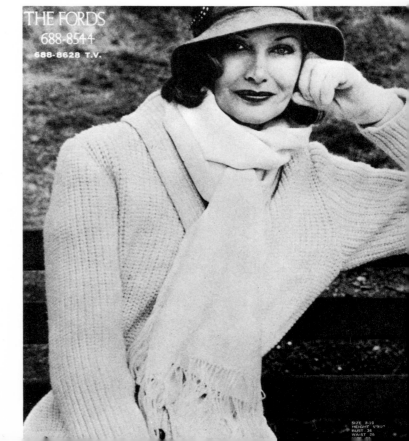

9. *How do you care for your hair?*
   Wash it once a week, put in balsam or other conditioner. It is colored every three weeks.
10. *What do you do to keep happy and interested in the world?*
   Always look at the bright side and alert yourself to what is going on in the world and around you in your daily life.
11. *Do you mind saying how old you are for publication?*
   In my beautiful forties.
12. *Do you have what you consider a coordinated beauty and/or health program?*
   Routine care and a special pamper day for beauty.
13. *Have you had or would you consider plastic surgery?*
   At the moment no.
14. *How do you feel about what is called "middle age"?*
   No such thing.

Betty Cornell Huston

1. *What years did you model?*
   1941–1960
2. *How many children do you have?*
   Three—twenty-one-year-old twins, boy and girl, Betsy and Jack; fourteen-year-old girl, Connie.
3. *Have you any grandchildren?*
   No.
4. *What were your weight and measurements as a model?*
   90 pounds; 30–18–30.
5. *What are your measurements today?*
   97 pounds; 32–23–33.
6. *Do you diet? If so, how?*
   No, but I do refrain from between-meal snacks, fried foods and rich desserts.
7. *How do you care for your skin?*
   I use moisturizer daily and avoid the direct rays of the sun.
8. *Do you exercise? If so, how often and how long?*
   No formal exercise; play golf and bowl weekly in season.

9. *How do you care for your hair?*
   I have my hair washed and set professionally weekly; have never resorted to hair dyes.
10. *What do you do to keep happy and interested in the world?*
   Wrote teen-age advice books and teen-age lectures up until ten years ago. Do volunteer work, enjoy taking care of my family. At present I am taking college courses.
11. *Do you mind saying how old you are for publication?*
   I was born April 14, 1927.
12. *Do you have what you consider a coordinated beauty and/or health program?*
   No.
13. *Have you had or would you consider plastic surgery?*
   No. I have never had plastic surgery. I would only consider plastic surgery in case of accident or disfigurement.
14. *How do you feel about what is called "middle age"?*
   What's "middle age"? It doesn't bother me at all.

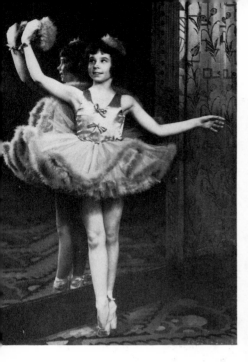

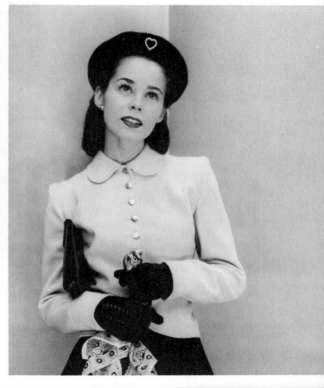

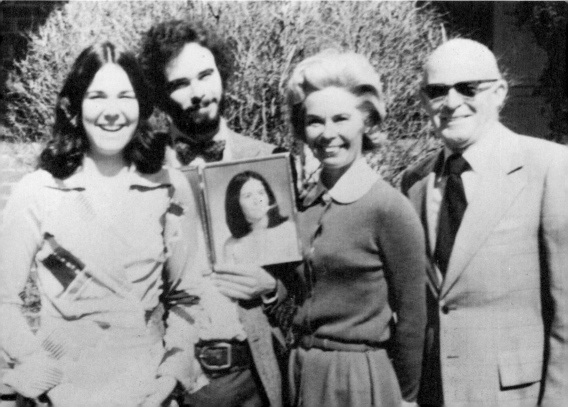

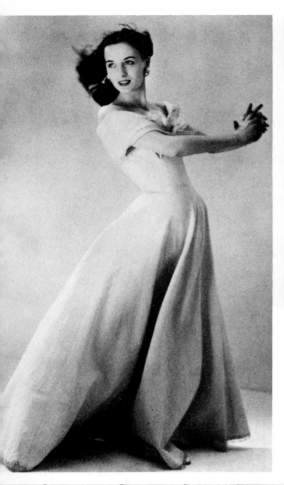
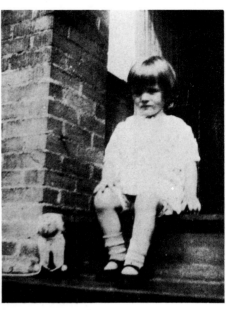
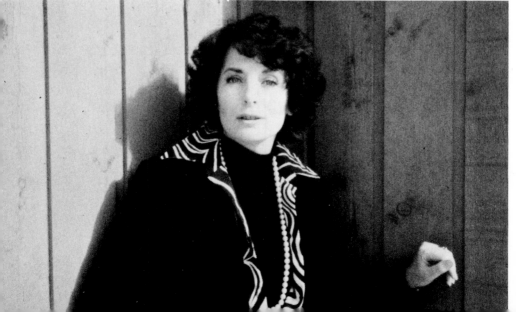

Lucille Lewis

1. *What years did you model?*
   1945–1952.
2. *How many children do you have?*
   Five.
3. *Have you any grandchildren?*
   Four.
4. *What were your measurements as a model?*
   34–24–35; 5 feet 8 inches.
5. *What are your measurements today?*
   34–25½–35½.
6. *Do you diet? If so, how?*
   Yes. Health foods, organic meats.
7. *How do you care for your skin?*
   No soap or sun on face, cleansing cream and night cream.
8. *Do you exercise? If so, how often and how long?*
   Yes, three times weekly, one to one and a half hours.
9. *How do you care for your hair?*
   Hairdressers.

10. *What do you do to keep happy and interested in the world?*
   Painting and sports.
11. *Do you mind saying how old you are for publication?*
   Forty-seven.
12. *Do you have what you consider a coordinated beauty and/or health program?*
   Yes.
13. *Have you had or would you consider plastic surgery?*
   Yes; ears when I was nineteen. I will consider other plastic surgery when necessary.
14. *How do you feel about what is called "middle age"?*
   A period for reevaluation to develop whatever potentials may have been submerged due to past responsibilities.

Romaine Simonson Maloney

1. *What years did you model?*
   1951–1957.
2. *How many children do you have?*
   Two boys.
3. *Have you any grandchildren?*
   No.
4. *What were your weight and measurements as a model?*
   110 pounds; 33–20–33½; 5 feet 7½ inches.
5. *What are your measurements today?*
   Same.
6. *Do you diet? If so, how?*
   Yes, by not eating very much.
7. *How do you care for your skin?*
   Soap and water. Moisturizer.
8. *Do you exercise? If so, how often and how long?*
   Yoga every day—one hour.
9. *How do you care for your hair?*
   Shampoo twice a week.

10. *What do you do to keep happy and interested in the world?*
Yoga is a very steadying force in my life. Plus, three years ago, I started a floor- and furniture-painting business, which is slowly beginning to get going.

11. *Do you mind saying how old you are for publication? If so, don't answer.*
Forty-three.

12. *Do you have what you consider a coordinated beauty and/or health program?*
Yoga.

13. *Have you had or would you consider plastic surgery?*
Have not had, and am not considering it.

14. *How do you feel about what is called "middle age"?*
It is a very challenging time of my life. The boys are going their way and it is necessary for me to restructure my life. Sometimes it's hard, but I'm optimistic and love the challenge!

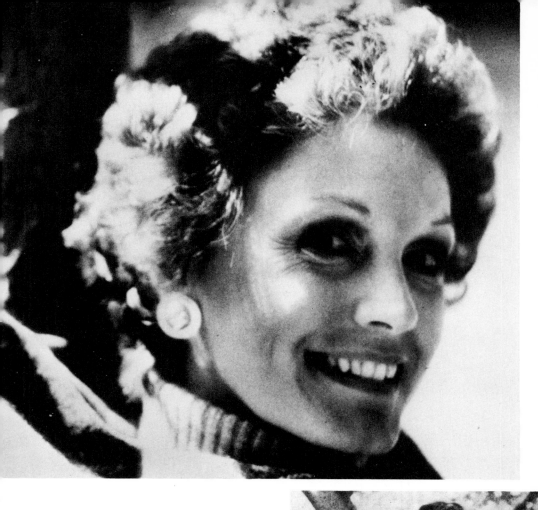

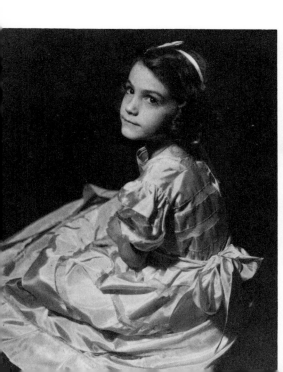

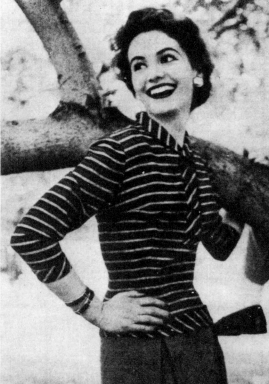

Jinx Falkenburg McCrary

1. *What years did you model?*
   From 1938 on.
2. *How many children do you have?*
   Two boys.
3. *Have you any grandchildren?*
   No.
4. *What were your weight and measurements as a model?*
   5 feet 8 inches; 130 pounds.
5. *What are your measurements today?*
   Approximately the same.
6. *Do you diet? If so, how?*
   High-protein, low-carbohydrate diet; weigh in each morning before breakfast to see if I am maintaining weight.
7. *How do you care for your skin?*
   Cleanse face at night with soap and water after removing makeup with removers; lubricate skin.
8. *Do you exercise? If so, how often and how long?*
   Walks each day; golf or tennis every day.

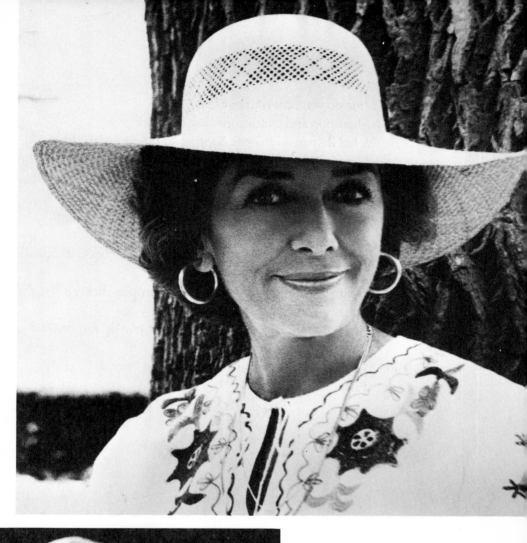

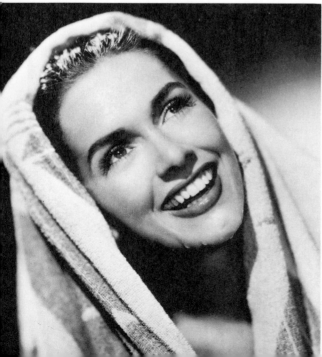

9. *How do you care for your hair?*
   Shampoo and conditioner once a week.
10. *What do you do to keep happy and interested in the world?*
    Have a "plan" for each day; avoid idle time; active in the North Shore University Hospital by serving as chairman of the associate trustees.
11. *Do you mind saying how old you are for publication?*
    No, fifty-seven.
12. *Do you have what you consider a coordinated beauty and/or health program?*
    Regular exercise and lots of it; proper diet and eight hours' sleep each night.
13. *Have you had or would you consider plastic surgery?*
    No, not yet.
14. *How do you feel about what is called "middle age"?*
    Fine.

Dina Merrill

1. *What years did you model?*

   I modeled for Vogue magazine and Vogue photographers for over a period of one year in the mid-forties, while I was going to drama school.

2. *How many children do you have?*

   I have three children.

3. *Have you any grandchildren?*

   No.

4. *What were your weight and measurements as a model?*

   My weight then varied between 117 pounds and 123 pounds.

5. *What are your measurements today?*

   123 pounds. I don't know what my measurements are exactly, but I know my waist and chest are both bigger today.

6. *Do you diet? If so, how?*

   No, I don't diet. However, I don't push my luck, and I eat very few rich desserts and pastries.

7. *How do you care for your skin?*
   Cleansing, moisturizing and protection from the sun.
8. *Do you exercise? If so, how often and how long?*
   Not the setting-up kind; but I do play tennis, golf, swim and ski.
9. *How do you care for your hair?*
   Once a week at the beauty parlor and streaks whenever needed, usually every six months.
10. *What do you do to keep happy and interested in the world?*
    I am an actress, I garden, do my sports, try to keep up with my children, and work for diabetic organizations throughout the country.
11. *Do you mind saying how old you are for publication?*
    Pass.
12. *Do you have what you consider a coordinated beauty and/or health program?*
    Not really. I try to take good care of my skin in the manner mentioned above, eat a good nutritious diet and get enough sleep.
13. *Have you had or would you consider plastic surgery?*
    Pass.
14. *How do you feel about what is called "middle age"?*
    It comes to all of us.

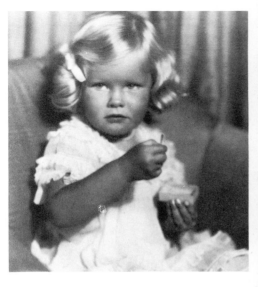

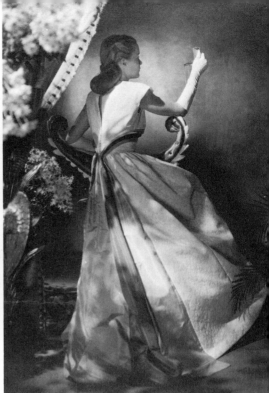

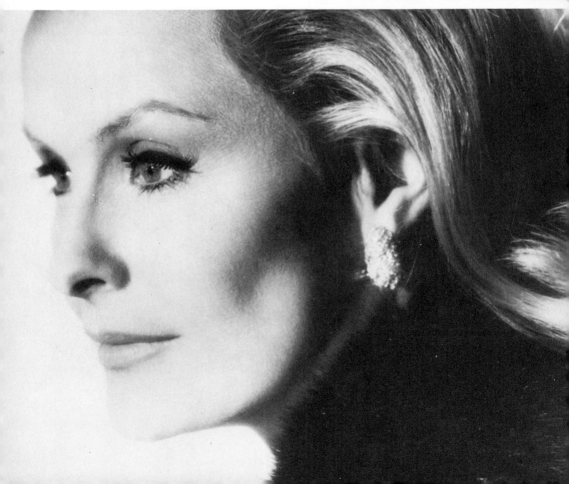

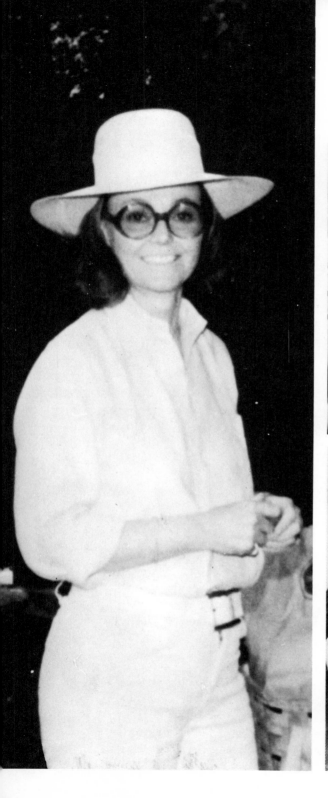

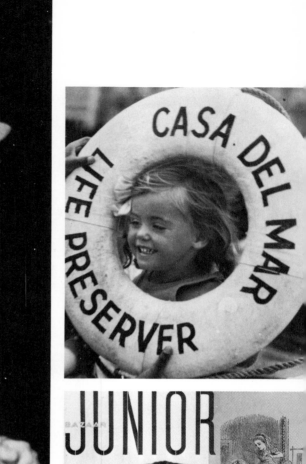

CASA DEL MAR
LIFE PRESERVER

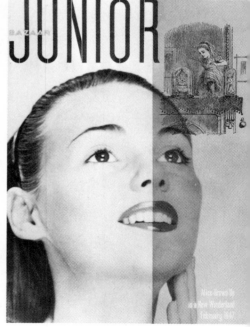

JUNIOR
BAZAAR

Pat Geoghegan Munn

1. *What years did you model?*
   1946–1966.
2. *How many children do you have?*
   One boy and one girl—son, twenty-two, daughter, twenty-four.
3. *Have you any grandchildren?*
   No.
4. *What were your measurements as a model?*
   5 feet 6 inches; 33–23–34.
5. *What are your measurements today?*
   34–26–36.
6. *Do you diet? If so, how?*
   Protein diet.
7. *How do you care for your skin?*
   Soap and water; creams.
8. *Do you exercise? If so, how often and how long?*
   Paddle tennis, bicycle, ski and walk a mile a day (at least).
9. *How do you care for your hair?*
   Wash twice a week.

10. *What do you do to keep happy and interested in the world?*
My own firm with partner, Timmins–Munn Associates. Interior designer.

11. *Do you have what you consider a coordinated beauty and/or health program?*
At least eight hours of sleep a day, eat properly.

12. *Have you had or would you consider plastic surgery?*
I think I would consider surgery if necessary, but I just grow old gracefully and don't need it.

13. *How do you feel about what is called "middle age"?*
State of mind! If you keep busy and don't let yourself go, there is no middle age. I loved modeling. It's the greatest career for a woman before she settles down to having children.

Lisa Fonsegrieves Penn

1. *What years did you model?*
   1934–1957.
2. *How many children do you have?*
   One girl, one boy.
3. *Have you any grandchildren?*
   Not yet.
4. *What were your weight and measurements as a model?*
   118 pounds; 35–23–33; 5 feet 9 inches.
5. *What are your measurements today?*
   35–23–33.
6. *Do you diet? If so, how?*
   No. I never sit still except at the movies.
7. *How do you care for your skin?*
   Soap and water. Eye cream on lids in small amount twice a day or more. Lots of fresh air, not too much sun.
8. *Do you exercise? If so, how often and how long?*
   Yes, every day, for ten minutes, swimming when possible, yoga.

9. *How do you care for your hair?*
Shampoo twice a week, followed by hair conditioner for
five minutes. Roll up under a scarf till dry. I never use
curlers, only hairpins very loosely set.

10. *What do you do to keep happy and interested in the world?*
I am a sculptor and intensely interested in the arts. Take
care of my family and share their problems and interests.
Love reading, music, film, people, travel, and hard work.

11. *Do you mind saying how old you are for publication? If so,
don't answer.*
As old as I look and as old as I feel. I never count the
years.

12. *Do you have what you consider a coordinated beauty
and/or health program?*
Only as previously stated. I'm a fresh-air addict. I think
love and work are the best beauty cares.

13. *Have you had or would you consider plastic surgery?*
Not now. I feel very much loved as I am. But who knows
about some thirty years from now.

14. *How do you feel about what is called "middle age"?*
Great! The best age so far.

15. *Did I leave out anything?*
Yes, I'm passionately in love with life.

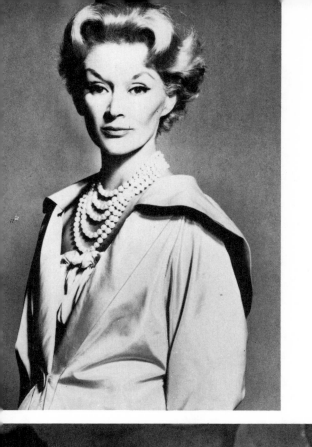
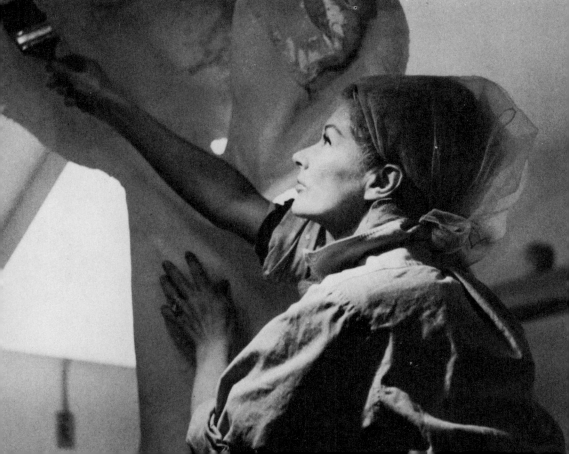

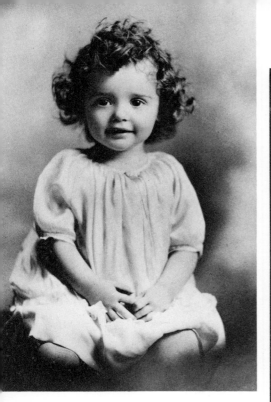

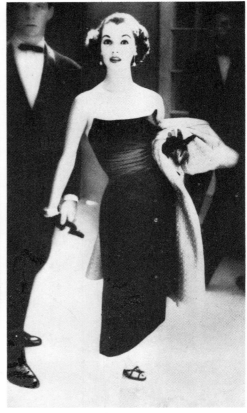

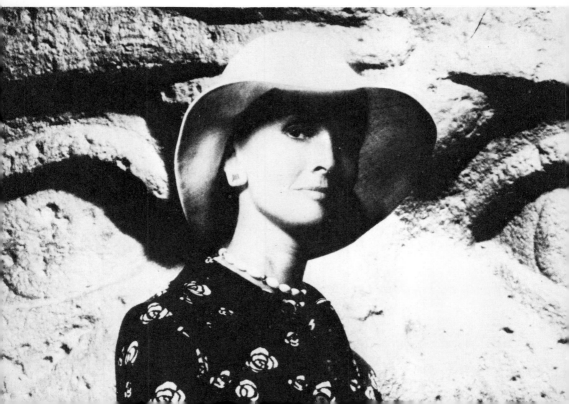

Nan Rees

1. *What years did you model?*
   1949–1961.
2. *How many children do you have?*
   Three.
3. *Have you any grandchildren?*
   No.
4. *What were your weight and measurements as a model?*
   104 to 108 pounds; 5 feet 7 inches; 33½–21–33.
5. *What are your measurements today?*
   110–112 pounds; 34–23–34.
6. *Do you diet? If so, how?*
   Not really, but always aware of intake.
7. *How do you care for your skin?*
   Soap and water and moisturizer.
8. *Do you exercise? If so, how often and how long?*
   Yoga, a half-hour daily, if lucky.
9. *How do you care for your hair?*
   Nothing special; color, short cut, three washes per week.

10. *What do you do to keep happy and interested in the world?*
Many interests: Teach two days a week at American Museum of Natural History (teach public-school children in African Mammals and Man halls). Amateur ornithologist, sail, garden, scuba, ski, learning to fly, fishing nut, lucky to safari in Africa for one month yearly.

11. *Do you have what you consider a coordinated beauty and/or health program?*
Yoga.

12. *Have you had or would you consider plastic surgery?*
Yes.

13. *How do you feel about what is called "middle age"?*
Have never felt better, have never enjoyed myself more.

Lois Wideman

1. *What years did you model?*
   1952–1961.
2. *How many children do you have?*
   Two.
3. *Have you any grandchildren?*
   No.
4. *What were your weight and measurements as a model?*
   110–115 pounds; 32–23–33; 5 feet 7 inches.
5. *What are your weight and measurements today?*
   115 pounds; 32–23–33.
6. *Do you diet? If so, how?*
   No.
7. *How do you care for your skin?*
   Nothing special—use a loofah mitt once or twice a week.
8. *Do you exercise? If so, how often and how long?*
   During summer, play tennis at least four hours a week. Wintertime play paddle tennis almost daily, ski occasionally, skate once a week. When in Florida, I swim daily.

9. *How do you care for your hair?*

Because it is very fine, I wash it two or three times a week with a mild shampoo. Blunt cut. And for special occasions, back to old-fashioned formula of beer for body.

10. *What do you do to keep happy and interested in the world?*

Am trial judging for USFSA [U.S. Figure Skating Association], was test chairman at a local skating rink, work for two charities, head of the volunteer library committee at Rumson Country Day School, paint; come summer, I accompany my daughter, KC, to weekly horse shows while she rides (and I hide my eyes!).

11. *Do you mind saying how old you are for publication? If so, don't answer.*

Will be forty-four this June.

12. *Do you have what you consider a coordinated beauty and/or health program?*

No, but hope springs eternal, and since my son, Fell, is off to prep school this fall, I sincerely am going to try to organize some sort of helpful regime.

13. *Have you had or would you consider plastic surgery?*

Why not? But I am a true coward re the knife and needle —anywhere! Seriously, I think it most beneficial, but I'd be just too chicken.

14. *How do you feel about what is called "middle age"?*

Aside from the statistic of my birth date, I feel physically much as I did when I was twenty-five. Emotionally I feel much more secure, but I'm not sure I know what all the fuss re middle age is about. (I suspect that if my kiddos were out of college and on their own, their absence in my daily life would leave a gap, thereby necessitating a reevaluation of my priorities.) But until that plateau arises, or other unforeseen conditions come to the fore, I truly don't consider middle age much more than a statistic garnered for data banks. (Boy! For someone who doesn't have many thoughts on the subject, I sure can rattle on!)

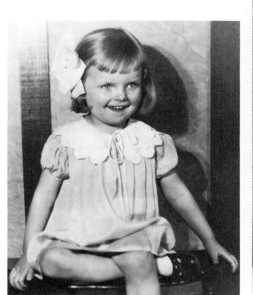

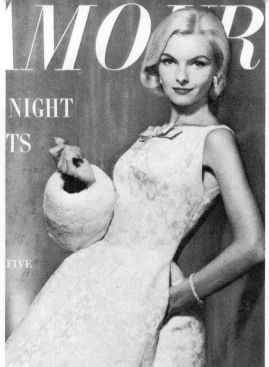

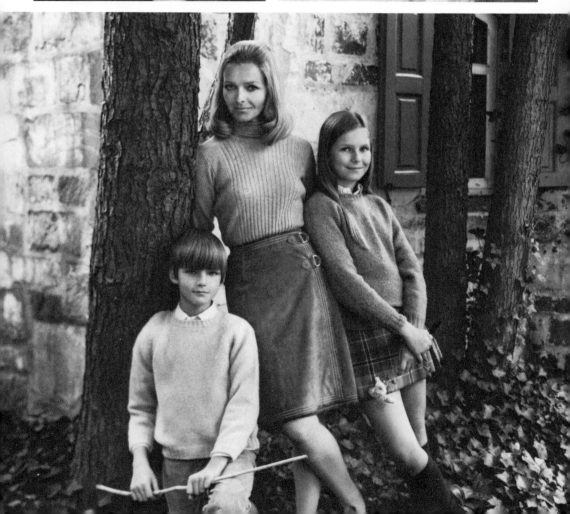

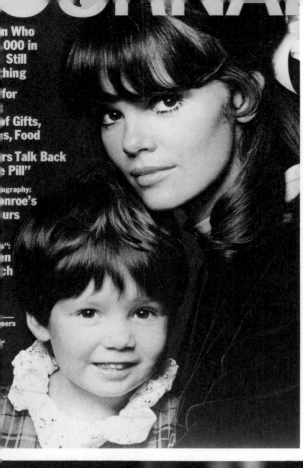

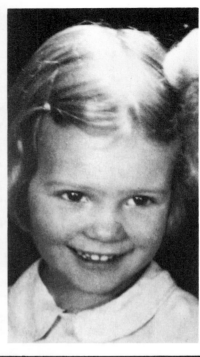

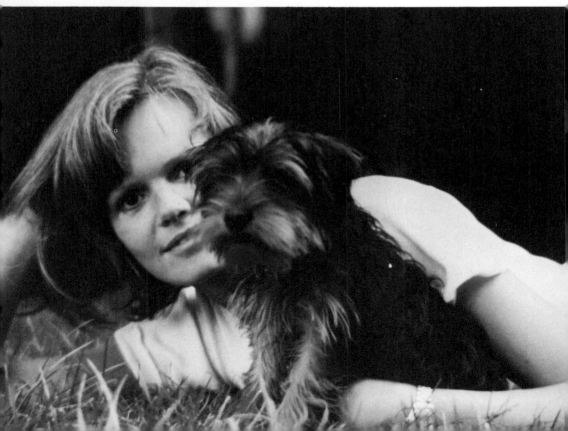

Marola Witt

1. *What years did you model?*
   About 1959 to 1972.
2. *How many children do you have?*
   Two.
3. *Have you any grandchildren?*
   No.
4. *What were your weight and measurements as a model?*
   I am 5 feet 9 inches. I weighed about 110 to 115 pounds.
5. *What are your measurements today?*
   I don't know my measurements but I do know that I weigh about twelve pounds more, meaning 120 to 124 pounds.
6. *Do you diet? If so, how?*
   No. Fortunately I do not need to diet; the extra weight I have put on, I needed.
7. *How do you care for your skin?*
   I keep it very clean, and day and night I use a cream, since I have very dry skin.

8. *Do you exercise? If so, how often and how long?*
   I play tennis twice a week and ski in the winter.
9. *How do you care for your hair?*
   I have it colored since I am gray, and I keep it shorter than I used to—this suits me better now that I am older.
10. *What do you do to keep happy and interested in the world?*
   I do all the things I did not do while I was working. But when the children reach sixteen or eighteen years, I'll want to go back to work (not modeling of course). Most girls, when they get married and have children, feel trapped and cooped up staying at home and are anxious to find something interesting to do. Not *me!* I love being home and not worrying about commuting, being on time, trying to juggle house, kids, dinner appointments, commitments for the children, for myself, for my husband, etcetera, with working. I can finally sit back and enjoy myself without being harried and hassled.
11. *Do you mind saying how old you are for publication? If so, don't answer.*
   I don't really mind, but ten years from now I might, at which time I might want to be younger, and anyone could prove me wrong if you want me to tell my age now. I can say this much—most people think I am older than I really am because I have such old children, both of whom were born when I was under twenty.
12. *Do you have what you consider a coordinated beauty and/or health program?*
   Not really.
13. *Have you had or would you consider plastic surgery?*
   Yes. Progress has been made in so many ways and the old-fashioned face-lift is a thing of the past. So many small things can be done to improve one's looks.
14. *How do you feel about what is called "middle age"?*
   I am looking forward to another era or stage. I worked very hard as a young girl; I was a mother when very young; and "middle age" means to me being independent again, with who knows what kind of career ahead of me.

WHY NOT YOU?

General Index

(An Index of Recipes follows)

in maintenance diet, 94
at health spas, *see* Spas
Breasts:
  attitudes toward, 153–54
  plastic surgery of, 153–56
  see also Mammaplasty
Brushing hair, 118–19
Buchinger Sanatorium (Bad Pyr-
    mont, Germany), 132
Buttocks, plastic surgery for,
    152–53

Calcium, 92
Calderone, Dr. Mary, 86
Carlson, Jane Cartwright, 190–
    193
Cancer, cryosurgery in treatment
    of, 151
Carbohydrates, in maintenance
    diet, 88–89
Cells, Virchow's research on, 139
Cell therapy, 139–41
Chagall, Marc, 135
Charles of the Ritz, 137, 138
Cheese, in maintenance diet, 93
Chemosurgery, 151
Chesnutt, Mme., 29
Childbearing, stretched muscles
    caused by, 85
Children, 180
  as means of meeting new
    people, 163–64
Chin:
  double, 149
  plastic surgery of, 149–50
Choline, 91
Churchill, Winston, 130
Circulation:
  exercises for, 104
  hair growth and, 118–19
Cleansing, *see* Bath; Shampoo;
    Skin care
Clinique Diététique (Cham-
    pigny, France), 139
Color rinse, 125
Craft, Jamie, 55
Crisco, for skin care, 112
Crisis years:
  defined, 19–20
  facing, planning for, 17–20
  see also Mental attitudes;
    Women

Cronin, Dr. Thomas D., 154
Cryosurgery, 151
Cuisinart, 173
Cyanacobalamin (B_{12}), 91

Dabney, Joanne, 39
Dandruff, 121
"Darling Charles," 55
David, Jack, 33
Dental work, and plastic surgery
    of chin, 149–50
Depression, 181
  see also Mental attitudes
Dermabrasion, 150
Deviated septum, surgery for, 148
Diaphragm, exercise for, 100
Diet:
  essential foods, 87–89
  Greenhouse menu, 138
  Maine Chance menu, 136–37
  minerals in, 92
  vitamin supplements, 92–93
  water in, 88–89
  see also Dieting; Interviews
    with models; Maintenance
    diet
Dieting:
  checking with doctor, 23–24
  exercises with, 23, 24, 63–66
  judging results, 23
  lunch when, 23
  menus for, 24–25, 28, 30, 32,
    35–36, 39, 42–43, 46, 49,
    51–52, 54, 56–57, 59, 61
  six rules for, 22–23
  small portions, 22
  vitamin C in, 23
  vitamin supplements while,
    92–93
  see also Fourteen-day diet;
    Interviews with models;
    Maintenance diet; Spas
Dietrich, Marlene, 108
Digestive system, vitamin B
    complex for, 90–91
Dillman, Suzy Parker, 47, 194–
    197
Diocles Carystos (Greek physi-
    cian), 134
Divorcees:
  problems of, 159, 160, 161

Ford, Billy, 19
Ford, Eileen, 29, 70
  attitude toward face-lift, 144
  books by, 17, 93, 95
  children, 19
  communication with women,
    182–83
  crisis years of, 19–20
  fourteen-day vegetarian diet,
    see Fourteen-day diet
  interviews with models, 187–
    243
  maintenance diet, 87–95
  personal use of makeup, 106
  survey of women, 176–83
Ford, Ermine, 38
Ford, Jamie, 19
Ford, Jerry, 19, 70
Ford, Katie, 19
Ford, Lacey, 19
Formwalt, Florence Dornan, 184,
  201–03
Fourteen-day diet, 23–63, 95
  checking with doctor, 23–24
  exercises with, 23, 24, 63–66
  Gevral protein in, 23
  gourmet fare in, 22
  judging results, 23
  liquid intake, 21–22
  menus, 24–25, 28, 30, 32, 35–
    36, 39, 42–43, 46, 51–52,
    54, 56–57, 59, 61
  small portions, 22
  vitamin C in, 23
Frosting (hair), 126
Frown lines, removal of, 147
Fruits, in maintenance diet, 94

Gay, Riccardo, 59
Genital prolapse, surgery for, 85–
  86
Gerovital H3, curative properties
  of, 141–42
Gevral protein, 23
  see also Menus (fourteen-day
    diet)
Gish, Lillian, 142
Glucose, 88–89
Golden Door (spa, Escondido,
  Calif.), 139
Grace, Princess of Monaco, 51
Graham, Karen, 28

Grapefruit juice, see Menus, four-
  teen-day diet
Gray hair, 122–23
Greenhouse, The (spa, Arlington,
  Texas), 137–39
  special services, 139
Grief, how to handle, 167–68
Griffin, Sunny, 62, 204–06
Griffith, Melanie, 34
Groueff, Lillian Fox, 207–09
"G.W.F., Jr.," 57

Hair, dyed or colored:
  aniline dyes, 125
  black dye, disadvantages of,
    124
  care and conditioning, 122–26;
    see also Hair care
  choosing a color, 123–24
  extra care, 126
  frosting as alternative, 126
  henna, 123–24, 125
  one-step dyeing, 125
  protection from sunlight, 123
  rinses, color shampoos, 125
  two-step dyeing, 126
Hairbrush, 118
Hair care, 117–29
  bristle brush for, 118–19
  conditioning, 119–21
  damaged, 121
  dandruff, 121
  dyed or colored, 122–26; see
    also Hair, dyed or colored
  gray, 122–23
  hairdresser's role, 128
  scalp massage, 118–19, 121
  shampooing, 119
  thinning hair, 121–22
  see also Interviews with models
Hairdresser, 128
Hair loss, 121–22
Hairpieces, 129
Hair straightening, 126–27
Hairstyle:
  choosing, 117–18, 127–28
  wigs and hairpieces, 128–29
Hamel, Veronica, 50
Hamilton, Alana, 26
Hamilton, George, 60
Harnett, Sunny:

One-minute exercises, 63–66,
96–98
see also Exercises
Orentreich, Dr. Norman, 122,
151–52
Oriental dancing, exercises based
on, 76–78
Ory, Iris, 37
Otopeni, Rumania, Dr. Aslan's
clinics at, 142
Otte, Loretta, 54

Parents Without Partners, 163–
164
Parker, Suzy, *see* Dillman, Suzy
Parker
Pelvis, exercises for flexibility, 73,
78–81, 83, 85
Penn, Lisa Fonsegrieves, 41–42,
231–33
Phosphorus, 92
Piazzi, Signora, 48
Pitanguy, Dr. Ivan, 152–53, 154,
155
Plastic surgery:
for abdomen, 153
attitudes toward, 144–45; *see
also* Interviews with models
for body defects, 152–56
for breasts, 153–55; *see also*
Mammaplasty
for buttocks, 152–53
for chin, 149–50
choosing a surgeon, 156
and dental work, 149–50
for ears, 150
for eyelids (blepharoplasty),
146–47
face-lift, 145–46
new techniques, 150–52
of nose (rhinoplasty), 147–49
for overhanging flesh above
eyes, 111
silicone, pros and cons, 147,
149, 151–52, 153–55
of vagina, 85–86
Politics, as opportunity for making friends, 165–66
Pontificia Universidade Católica
(Rio de Janeiro, Brazil), 152
Pope Pius XII, cured by Dr.
Aslan, 141

Popov, Dr. Ivan, 140–41
Potassium, 92
Prairie, La, *see* La Prairie
Protein:
Gevral, 23
in maintenance diet, 87
Psychological techniques, for
changing mental attitudes,
168–69
Pyridoxine (B_6), 90–91

Rees, Dr. Thomas, 152
Rees, Nan, 40, 234–36
Renaissance (spa, Nassau, Ba-
hamas), 140–41
Rhinoplasty (plastic surgery of
nose), 147–49
Rhytidectomy (face-lift), *see*
Face-lift
Riboflavin (B_2), 90
Rinses, color, 125

Salads, in maintenance diet,
93–94
Salt:
and water retention, 89
herbs in place of, 89–90
Salt-free diet, sodium in, 92
San Blas (Indian spa, Nayarit,
Mexico), 131
Saratoga, N.Y., mineral baths at,
131
Scalp:
conditioning, massage, 118–21
dandruff, 121
see also Thinning hair
Scarlett, Katie, 57
School, for extending social and
intellectual life, 159–60
Schulte, Lily, 37
Self-awareness, 171–75
test for, 172–74
see also Mental attitudes
Sex:
exercises to improve mobility,
performance, 71–86
fatigue and, 70
femininity and, 68
initiation by woman, 70
lifelong need for, 69–70, 71

male attitudes, 68, 69
in middle years and beyond,
  71, 86
importance to relationships,
  67–68
revitalization of sex life, 71–72
survey of women on, 179
Sexual mobility, exercises for,
  71–86
Sexual problems, Gerovital H3
  for, 142
Sexual responsiveness, 68–69
Shampoo, shampooing, 119
  color shampoo, 125
Shrimpton, Jean, 46
SIECUS (Sex Information and
  Education Council of U.S.),
  86
Silicone:
  in breast surgery, 153–55
  in facial surgery, 151–52
  for nose buildup, 149
  for removing frown lines,
    wrinkles, 147
Skin:
  plastic surgery for blemishes,
    150–52
  see also Skin care
Skin care, 111–14
  for adult acne, 112, 114
  astringents and toners, 112–13
  basic principles, 112
  bath, 114–16
  evening, 113–14
  moisturizing, 113
  morning, 112
  vitamin A for, 90
  weekly facial, 114
  see also Interviews with
    models; Makeup
Snacks, in maintenance diet, 95
Snagov clinic (Dr. Aslan's), 142
Soap, for skin care, 112
Sodium, 92
"Soni C.," 63
Spas for health and beauty, 130–
  143
  Bad Pyrmont, 132
  Beauty Farm, 139
  Bircher-Benner Sanatorium,
    132–34
  Buchinger Sanatorium, 132

cell therapy at, 139–41
Clinique Diététique, 139
foods used for healing, 132–34
Golden Door, The, 139
Greenhouse, The, 137–39
Institute for Geriatrics, 142
La Prairie, 130, 140
Maine Chance, 135–37
mineral-bath-oriented, 131–32
at Otopeni, Rumania, 142
Renaissance, 140–41
San Blas ("sand pack cure"),
  131
Snagov clinic, 142
Spier, Corinne, 52
Spine, limbering exercise for,
  78–79
Spry, for skin care, 112
Straightening hair, 126–27
Strandgaard, Birte, 62
Subconscious, and changing
  mental attitudes, 168–69
Submandibular lipectomy, for
  double chin, 149
Survey of Women, Eileen Ford's,
  176–83
  boredom, 180
  children, 180
  depression, nervousness, 181
  drinking, 180–81
  husbands, women's likes and
    dislikes in, 177–78, 179, 180
  income, age range, 176
  marriage, 176–77, 181; see also
    subentry above, husbands
  mutual interests, 179–80
  new problems, 182
  sex, sex relations, 179
Sugar, 88–89
  in maintenance diet, 94
Suppleness, all-over exercises for,
  76–78
Surgery, see Plastic surgery

Teeth:
  calcium for, 92
  correction of, as adjunct to fa-
    cial surgery, 149–50
  vitamins for, 90, 91
Teflon pan, 93
Thiamine (B_1), 90

Index of Recipes

Endive with watercress salad,
49–50
Eggplant:
appetizer al Papacito Martin,
50
ratatouille cappucine, 26
sautéed, 59–60
slices, baked, 32
soufflé–Darling Charles, 55

Fried cabbage–Loretta Otte, 54
Fried parsley served all over
Paris, 33–34
French dressing, 25–26
see also Vinaigrette sauce

Galya Milovskaya's blender
borscht, 29
Gazpacho, blender, 47
Ghivetch, Rumanian, 41
Green bean salad, 27
Green beans–Ali MacGraw, 35
Grilled tomatoes–Ewa Karrlan-
der, 60

Hearts of palm with anchovy
dressing–Joanne Dabney,
39–40
Herb dressing (for chicory and
orange salad), 42
Hollandaise, blender, 60

Italian spinach–Elsa Martinelli,
45
Italian spinach–Soni C., 63

Jamie Craft's salad, 55

Lala's salade de romaine, 30–31
Leeks, puree of, 29
Lettuce:
braised, 45
with melted margarine–Katie
Scarlett, 57
see also Salads

Mashed winter squash–Mikael
Katz, 53
Menus (fourteen-day diet):
Day 1, 24–25
Day 2, 28

Day 3, 30
Day 4, 32–33
Day 5, 35–36
Day 6, 39
Day 7, 42–43
Day 8, 46
Day 9, 49
Day 10, 51–52
Day 11, 54
Day 12, 56–57
Day 13, 59
Day 14, 61
Mint and orange salad, 46
Mixed vegetable grill–Sunny
Griffin, 62
Mixed vegetable dishes:
ghivetch, 41
ratatouille cappucine, 26
vegetable grill, 62
see also Salads; specific vege-
table names
Mozzarella, tomato and basil
salad, 59–60
Muesli (grain-and-fruit health
food), 132–33
Mushrooms:
broiled, stuffed, 53
champignons à la grecque, 52
in mixed vegetable grill, 62
salade de champignons, 28
sautéed, 44
Mushroom salad–Birte Strandgaard, 62
Mushroom sauce with artichoke
bottoms, 40
Mushroom and zucchini casserole, 34

Orange and chicory salad with
herb dressing, 41–42
Orange and mint salad–Jean
Shrimpton, 46

Panama consommé, 26
Parsley, fried, 33–34
Peppers, sautéed, 29–30
Puree of broccoli–Tippi Hedren,
32
Puree of leeks–Eileen's favorite,
29

Ratatouille cappucine, 26
Red cabbage with apples—Trice
    Tomsen, 48–49
Red cabbage—Senta Berger, 38
Romaine salad with anchovies
    and cheese, 30–31
Roquefort dressing (for lettuce),
    43
Rumanian ghivetch à la Nina
    Blanchard, 41

Salad(s)
    Boston lettuce with Roquefort
        dressing, 43
    chef's, 32
    chicory and orange, 41–42
    Jamie Craft's (raw and cooked
        vegetables), 55
    mixed (vegetables, greens), 25
    mushroom, 28, 62
    orange and mint, 46
    romaine, with anchovies,
        cheese, 30–31
    salade de champignons, 28
    string bean, 27
    tomato, mozzarella, basil,
        59–60
    Trini's Sardinian (eggs, cheese,
        romaine), 44
    watercress and endive, 49–50
Salad—Lauren Hutton (mixed
    vegetables, greens), 25
Salad dressings:
    anchovy, 39–40
    anchovy and beet, 57
    French, 25–26
    herb (for chicory-orange
        salad), 42
    Roquefort, 43
    for Trini's Sardinian salad, 44
    for watercress-endive salad, 50
    see also Vinaigrette sauce
Salade de champignons—Karen
    Graham, 28
Sauces:
    blender hollandaise, 60
    mushroom (with artichoke
        bottoms), 60
    vinaigrette, 36–37, 47, 52–53
    see also Salad dressings
Sautéed eggplant slices—Ric-
    cardo Gay, 59–60

Sautéed peppers—Jolly Earl,
    29–30
Sautéed mushrooms—Maude
    Adams, 44
Sliced tomatoes with anchovy
    and beet dressing—G.W.F.,
    Jr., 57
Soups:
    blender borscht, 29
    blender gazpacho, 47
    Panama consommé, 26
Spinach:
    Italian, 45, 63
    with pignolis, 55
    rings, with carrots, 51
    in stuffed tomatoes, 31
    with tomatoes, 29
Spinach à la Jennifer O'Neill, 55
Spinach rings with carrots—
    Princess Grace of Monaco,
    51
Spinach-stuffed tomatoes—Susan
    Blakely, 31
Spinach with tomatoes—Mme.
    Chesnutt, 29
Squash:
    mashed winter, 53
    see also Zucchini
Steamed broccoli with blender
    hollandaise—George Hamil-
    ton, 60
Steamed broccoli—Veronica
    Hamel, 50
Stewed tomatoes—Kay Bourland,
    56
String bean salad—Candice
    Bergen, 27
Stuffed zucchini—Iris Ory, 37

Tomato, mozzarella and basil
    salad—Parco dei Principi,
    59–60
Tomatoes:
    creole, 38
    with cucumber ice, 61–62
    grilled, with sour cream, 60
    in mixed vegetable grill, 62
    sliced, with anchovy-beet
        dressing, 57
    spinach-stuffed, 31
    stewed, 56

Tomatoes creole à la Ermine
Ford, 38
Tomatoes with cucumber ice—
Inger Malmeroos, 61–62
Trini's Sardinian salad with
dressing, 44

Vegetable(s)
grill, 62
mixed, *see* Mixed vegetables
stew (ghivetch), 41
see also Salads; specific
vegetables
Vinaigrette sauce:
for artichokes, 47

for artichokes with asparagus,
36–37
for cold asparagus, 52–53

Watercress and endive salad—
Ann Turkel, 49–50

Zucchini:
and mushroom casserole, 34
in a pan, 48
ratatouille cappucine, 26
stuffed, 37
Zucchini and mushroom casserole
—Melanie Griffith, 34
Zucchini in a pan alla Signora
Piazzi, 48